D1075041

37653003958868
Southwest
612.821 A
Sleep and its secrets : the
river of crystal light

✓

**CENTRAL ARKANSAS
LIBRARY SYSTEM
SOUTHWEST
BRANCH LIBRARY**
LITTLE ROCK, ARKANSAS

JUL 17 1996
DEMCO

Sleep and Its Secrets

The River of Crystal Light

Sleep and Its Secrets

The River of Crystal Light

Michael S. Aronoff, M.D.

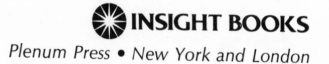

INSIGHT BOOKS

Plenum Press • New York and London

Library of Congress Cataloging-in-Publication Data

Aronoff, Michael S.
    Sleep and its secrets : the river of crystal light / Michael S.
  Aronoff.
       p.   cm.
    "Insight books."
    Includes bibliographical references and index.
    ISBN 0-306-43968-9
    1. Sleep.   I. Title.
    [DNLM: 1. Sleep.   WL 108 A769s]
  QP425.A76   1991
  154.6--dc20
  DNLM/DLC
  for Library of Congress   91-24100
                                                                       CIP

Cover photo by Michael S. Aronoff, M.D.

ISBN 0-306-43968-9

© 1991 Plenum Press, New York
A Division of Plenum Publishing Corporation
233 Spring Street, New York, N.Y. 10013

An Insight Book

All rights reserved

No part of this book may be reproduced, stored in a retrieval system, or transmitted
in any form or by any means, electronic, mechanical, photocopying, microfilming,
recording, or otherwise, without written permission from the Publisher

Printed in the United States of America

CENTRAL ARKANSAS LIBRARY SYSTEM
SOUTHWEST BRANCH
LITTLE ROCK, ARKANSAS

To the memory of my father, William R. Aronoff,
and to my daughters, Amanda and Jessica.
They have anchored me, and are an inspiration
to me . . . more than he knew or they know.

Prefatory Note

Wynken, Blynken and Nod one night
Set sail in a wooden shoe
Sailed on a river of crystal light
Into a sea of dew. . . .
Eugene Field,
Wynken, Blynken & Nod

The wellspring of this book actually derives from two sources. First, the fascination with human behavior and the mechanisms by which it is piloted. Secondly, the joy of adventure and discovery.

With regard to the first, consider this venture a guided expedition . . . not through the Amazon Rain Forest, along the Great Barrier Reef, nor round the limitless corridors of space, but closer. Much closer. Within us all, just over the boundary from wakefulness, and occupying fully one-third of our lives, lies a mysterious world both timed and timeless. This realm of sleep, with its rules, mechanisms, and inventions, and with its dreams, soundlessly whispering in our unguarded ears, is subject to vagaries which affect the very pulsing and throbbing of life itself. It is into this dominion that we sail.

Regarding the second fount from which this work springs, we shall be like travelers in a fascinating but foreign land . . . sharing the explorers' delights of discovery, carried along by interest and bolstered by the building knowledge about what we observe. Throughout, our curiosity will serve as a beacon to help illuminate the way as we embark on this journey down the "river of crystal light."

Acknowledgments

No endeavor, such as this project, reaches completion without the input, both direct and indirect, of many supporters. I am indebted to a large number of such colleagues, friends, and family. And I am now privileged to have a platform from which to express my appreciation and my gratitude, both of which have always been felt but perhaps not completely articulated.

With regard to my colleagues, they come in two forms. The first is my professional mentors and peers through whom I have been exposed to a level of intellectal discipline, sophistication, and challenge that was, and continues to be, extraordinary. They include Drs. Francis H. Parker, Eliot Stellar, Daniel X. Freedman, Willard Gaylin, Frederick K. Goodwin, Howard F. Hunt, Shervert H. Frazier, Roger A. Mackinnon, and Robert Michels . . . thoughtful teachers and superb researchers and clinicians who proved to be not only sources of seasoned knowledge but also of sage advice. A special acknowledgment to three colleagues, in particular: Dr. Leith McMurray, with whom I initiated preliminary discussions about this book many years ago, and Dr. Richard C. Friedman and Dr. Zira DeFries, stimulating and supportive friends through thick and thin.

The second group of colleagues comprises patients who provided me with the opportunity to know them and to grow with them. They must indeed be acknowledged.

I am grateful to two friends, especially, A. Joseph Lipton and

Caroline Edwards, who have generously and selflessly supported me and my endeavors. And to my editor, Norma Fox, whose iron hand never once showed through her silken glove, I am indebted for her faith and for her sensitive and gentle guidance. The three have much in common: they are all competent, full of insight and humor, and are never heavy-handed.

I must also acknowledge a man I have never met personally, but whose writing and breadth of interest exerted a profound influence on my own thinking and whose books provided me with the model for this one . . . Dr. Carl Sagan.

My parents, Reva and Bill, provided my brother and me with an atmosphere of humor, optimism, and intellectual curiosity. It has stood me in good stead and for it I will always be grateful. Finally, I want to thank my wife, Dara, for her loving support, editorial help, and understanding throughout this venture and through our lives together. I am indeed fortunate.

Contents

Chapter 1

Introduction

Sleep had been, until recently, the dark one-third of our lives and, like the far side of the moon, a persistent mystery for all humanity. As with all areas of mystery, it has become entangled with folklore and ritual. Known only indirectly through dimly remembered dreams and the drowsiness associated with falling asleep and awakening, sleep has always been linked with poetry, myth and time-honored superstition. None of us can study himself or herself while asleep nor converse with another who is asleep. But just as the space age has given us instruments to view the far side of the moon, nurturing a more sophisticated knowledge of our planetary environment, so too has it given us the means to investigate, in a far less speculative manner, aspects of brain function leading to a more sophisticated knowledge of our inner environment: Questions regarding the kinds of sleep we are subject to, the variation in the intensity of this sleep, and even the very purpose of sleep can now be entertained. And it is precisely because of everyone's "indirect" experience of it that sleep lends itself so well to an exposition of the power, validity, and fascination of a scientific approach to the understanding of a human activity.

But it has not always been so that we have even appreciated the fact that the seat of sleep resides in the brain. That pillar of Greek enlightenment, Aristotle, attributed to the heart, and anatomically located there, the function of sense perception and sleep. It was not until the 13th century, during the late Renaissance (according to a medical historian by the name of Dannenfeldt), that a philosopher named Albertus Magnus described the *brain* as the location where the vital spirit, derived from the heart, was "perfected," controlling the animal powers within and bringing about sensation and sleep.

Although interest in sleep and its problems has captivated all of us for years, much of what will be presented here is the result of more recent research. New information on nutrition and brain function, "chronobiology," differences in function between the left and right brain halves regarding thinking and dreaming, and new understanding of normal sleep patterns . . . all these are examples of recent developments that will shed new light on our appreciation of sleep phenomena. The intent of this book is to be more than just philosophically interesting; it is expected to be of help to anyone with questions about sleep-related phenomena or problems.

A HISTORICAL PERSPECTIVE

People often judge the quality of their day-to-day living by the quality of their sleep. Consider how frequently you will hear people explaining their current mood state by referring to how they slept the night before. What goes into judgments of such quality? Many factors are known to impact on the nature of sleep. These include physical factors (such as living conditions and external circumstances in the sleeping environment), psychological factors (such as personality types and level of stress), and physiological factors (such as diet, physical activity, and general state of health). Early medical theorists like the ancient Greek authorities of Galen and Hippocrates speculated about the effect of various sleep positions and theorized about the effect of various combinations and permutations of hot food, cold food, liquids and, of course, the heavenly bodies, on the kind and amount of sleep that a person could expect. What they did not speculate about was the underlying, organismic basis for sleep to begin with. Their perspective did not leave room for any question about the very physiological "engine" that might be driving the sleep phenomenon.

Aristotle refined the thinking of the day regarding the effects of external events on sleep and how the body physiology was dependent on sleep. It was he who first speculated about a mechanism for sleep. In his *Parva Naturalia*, he concluded that "evaporations" from the digestive system produced sleep, perhaps drifting upwards like the swirling mists of the opium den. In many ways, reasoning along the lines of sleep being a phenomenon not integral to the body's physiology but visited upon it from the outside had its beginnings in early prescriptions for the number and ingredients of meals and the positions to be assumed during sleep. For instance, in his 1562 treatise *Bulwarke of Defence againste all Sicknes, Somes, and Woundes*, William Bullein wrote,

> ". . . to lye upon the backe, with a gaping mouth, is dangerous: and many, thereby, are made starke ded in their sleepe; through apoplexia, and obstruction of the senews, of the places vitalle, animall, and nutrimentalle."

Another example of crediting external agents for the control of bodily processes can be seen in the writing of William Bailey, physician to Queen Elizabeth, who in *A Briefe Treatise Touching the Preservation of the Eiesight* in 1602, warned about sleeping in a room exposed to moonlight; such exposure, he opined, caused "rheumatic diseases." Incidentally, for all of these fascinating glimpses into the history of early medical speculation, I am indebted to the author Karl H. Dannenfeldt who, in 1986, published in the *Journal of the History of Medicine and Allied Sciences* an in-depth survey entitled "Sleep: Theory and Practice in the Late Renaissance." We do not have to look too far back into our past to note the popularity of the sleeping cap and then to see its antecedents in admonitions from the late 16th century that the head must be kept warm during sleep . . . but not too warm. Dannenfeldt quotes the 16th century physician Vaughan's caution that if the head is kept too warm, "the excess heat would astonish the minde and spirit."

MIND AND BRAIN: BOTH SIDES OF THE LOOKING GLASS

Sleep is a part of our lives, yet even today we have been in particular ignorance of it. Lewis Carroll used the metaphor of the Looking Glass, in Alice's adventures, to divide mental life into sleeping and waking segments, and, further, to explore the interface between the two. I propose to shift the emphasis and usage of this metaphor in order to explore the subjective–objective interface of "mind" and "brain." Just as there were strange apparitions in Alice's looking glass that became more comprehensible upon closer acquaintance, there are in our looking glass hitherto inexplicable forms, such as neurons and chemicals, taking on more comprehensible shape as our scientific familiarity with them increases. Because of a series of scientific advances on a multitude of fronts that bear on this very personal topic, it is timely to correlate these findings from diverse disciplines and to demystify the phenomenon of sleep. In the process, perhaps a renewed appreciation for the power of the scientific approach to issues regarding personal existence will be instilled. These findings may then be contrasted to the narrow, fad-bound attitudes that govern so much of what is written on personal health concerns today.

Those of us involved in the medical sciences recognize that a scientific attitude toward a topic, such as a health concern, still permits considerable scope for imagination and speculation. Yet for all that we might speculate about, we must submit to the discipline of distinguishing between what is known with reasonable certainty and what is merely plausible. Too many health cults have grown up around a few facts formed into logically consistent but empty formulae that prevent the growth of new knowledge. The pursuit of more knowledge and deeper understanding is the essence of the approach of medical science. That previous scientific formulations have proved inadequate is to be taken as a matter of course. The search for new facts and greater understanding is a never-ending endeavor, and enough new facts will always overthrow old, revered theories, scientific or otherwise. It is expressly because of the breathtaking pace at which new information is being discovered that this presentation is necessary—for the rate at which excellent scientific theories become old and moribund, sadly, like scientific books such as this, is accelerating. A scientific theory, like a politician's term in office, serves to coordinate all the extant facts of life for that particular moment in time. When the facts of life change, so must the theories and political leaders. Because of the new pace of discoveries, no single theory can last long.

Perhaps this is why cultism seems to have made increasing inroads of late. How comforting to know from the cradle to the grave that the sign of the zodiac controls your fate. Anyway, medical science has been proven "wrong" so many times; besides, these scientists are always changing their minds!

By presenting a series of interdependent modules, however, each surveying an aspect of the sleep phenomenon, I hope to demonstrate that control over one's own sleep and health is best achieved by opening oneself up to the wealth of new information that is flooding in. This presentation attempts to be a guide to this new information—an open-ended invitation to investigate and learn from a scientific perspective—rather than a close-cycle "how to" tract that purports to be the very last word and ultimate authority on the subject. If, after reading this, you find yourself more interested in learning new facts than in acquiring only a series of rituals to guide your sleep habits, my intentions will have been well served.

MODELS IN BIOLOGICAL PSYCHIATRY

This book breaks down the study of sleep into segments, each dealing with an aspect of sleep. In part, this is done in order to show how the investigation of an activity at different levels of inquiry can be integrated so as to yield a meaningful and practical perspective. And while the data and concepts to be discussed here are specifically related to sleep, the general framework also applies to the study of other biobehavioral phenomena.

We are about to provide structure to a phenomenon that exists in that middle ground between biology and psychology, and between biochemistry on a submicroscopic scale and evolution on a cosmic scale. Sleep is such a phenomenon. But even as we dissect and examine the sleep–wake cycle from a number of different perspectives, we are creating a representation, sculpting a form, from an inner, stable armature on out. Like the evolutionary paleontologist reconstructing his *papier mâché* model of a long-extinct dinosaur, we will apply strips of information from different sources and build up, layer by layer, an image, a model that incorporates our knowledge to date about sleep.

Models, simply, are theoretical creations developed to classify and give meaning to what has been observed or thought to exist. Any such proposal or model can rapidly become quite complex because, in the biological and psychological world of action and reaction, there are often several intermediary mechanisms in the chain reaction which begin with an environmental stimulus and result in the response of the organism to that stimulus. So, for example, an external stimulus (the presence of a predator) is perceived by the organism, say a deer. The perceiving organ, aided by its specialized organelles, transduces the information to a nervous impulse which is transmitted to central processing units in the brain, including, for instance, the hypothalamus (a particular neuronal grand junction from which chemical messengers, called polypeptides, are released). These messengers, once released, are sent to a central dispatching area (the pituitary gland) which is kicked into action, Rube Goldberg-like, first producing an energy- and manufacturing-facilitating compound known as cyclic AMP, and then triggering the release of agents known as trophic hormones. These chemicals wend their way to target cells in organs and glands elsewhere in the body, where, Paul Revere-like, they call out for the release of substances (such as adrenal steroids and epinephrine) which cause muscles to move, hearts to pound, and alarms to ring. Each one of these intermediary steps, in this example of a model of behavioral response, can additionally be seen as a buffer, insulating the entire system in a stepwise fashion to ensure both responsiveness and relative stability of the system despite the pressures and whims of an ever-changing environment.

When we talk of sleep and ask questions about its purpose, we will always (either directly or implicitly) be referring to some model representing our current understanding of the biology and psychology of the sleep–wake cycle. More specifically, questions like: What type of sleep should one have for effective waking performance? Does each stage of sleep meet a particular or unique need? What are the recuperative values of different kinds of sleep? Why is a brief nap refreshing for some? Why do some people remember their dreams? Why do some seem to avoid going to sleep? What are the effects of oversleeping or under-sleeping? These and many other questions are all viewed through, and then explicated within, a theoretical construct representing a view of human behavior. Models relevant to our study here focus on cause-and-effect relationships as well as buffering or "homeostatic" functions. Our discussion will interweave a number of these different attempts at explanation—or "models"—as we discuss various aspects of the phenomenon of sleep.

But another issue, relevant to all discussions about phenomena overlapping both the biological and the psychological domains, should be mentioned before we proceed further: I believe that there is a biological basis to behavior but that behavior is not controlled exclusively by biological factors. This may seem self-evident to some of you; however, in investigating the foundations of this control, there is always the difficulty in relating, for example, levels of brain chemicals (that go by names such as the catecholamines epinephrine and norepinephrine, and cyclic AMP) to the metabolism and activity of discrete yet interconnected clusters of neurons and the different psychological functions they facilitate. And, contrariwise, whatever components determine an individual's behavioral state at any one moment in time may alter the metabolism and thereby influence the physiological state upon which the particular phenomenon in question is being played out. Finally, the details of chemical effects on distinct aspects of behavioral response patterns can be quite difficult to discern, in part because important though small influences may simply be masked by "noise"—that is, by other ongoing reactions within the system which our investigational tools are still too undeveloped to detect. In the flow of continuing behavior, many different events occur at the same time and they can have resonating effects on each other. Under such circumstances, it is often difficult to know what correlates with what, let alone what is caused by what.

AN ARCHITECTURAL MODEL OF SLEEP

Before proceeding further, let us first describe the so-called architecture of sleep, that is, its typical component stages as they are distinguished from each other by their characteristic electroencephalographic (EEG) tracing signatures, and by their differential "depth" (or responsiveness to external stimuli). There are five such components, which can be further subdivided into two groups based on the presence or absence of rapid eye movements (REM): quick, darting movements of the eyes, coursing from side to side behind closed eyelids in the sleeping individual. Stages 1, 2, 3, and 4 are sleep components of increasing depth that occur sequentially, and in which REM are not observed. Consequently, they are referred to, collectively, as nonrapid eye movement (NREM) sleep. Stage 1 is the lightest and stage 4 is the deepest. A person is in stage 2 for about half of a total night's sleep. The sleep stage characterized by the presence of REM is the fifth component stage and is, by definition, the sleep stage in which REM are found. It is similar in depth to stage 2, and first occurs in a night's sleep about 90 minutes after a complete cycle of sleep stages 1 to 4 has been traversed.

REM sleep is also known as the dream state, the D state, or paradoxical sleep (this last, because the EEG suggests the presence of a type of brain cortex activation, even though the subject is asleep). It is further characterized by a virtual paralysis or disconnection of the muscular system, but a rise in the activity of the heart rate, respiratory system and the sexual organs, and by an increase in blood pressure as well. In addition to the aforementioned increase in activity of the muscles controlling eye movement, and the relative activation of brain electrical patterns as reflected by the sleep-EEG, REM sleep is notable for the occurrence of dreams. Although the mechanisms involved in the regulation of our observance of logic and reality in waking life are working at considerably reduced capacity during REM sleep, the degree of mental activation remains high. This is reflected in the operations necessary for dreaming to occur (including such functions as drawing from memory, perceptual recognition, and the ability to learn and commit to memory).

In contrast to the REM sleep unitary EEG profile, NREM sleep has four subdivisions, ranging from light sleep (stage 1) through to deep, Delta, or slow wave sleep (stage 4). Overall characterization of NREM sleep includes a picture reciprocal to that of REM sleep. In NREM sleep, one sees the preservation and maintenance of more muscle tone than in REM sleep, so that, although there may not be much in the way of overt motor action observable, the capacity for movement is more readily available.

This will have consequences that we will examine when we turn to discuss sleep disorders in Chapter 9. Coupled with this maintained level of muscle tone is a relative unresponsiveness to sensory stimuli. This results in an elevated arousal threshold which progresses as the depth of NREM sleep increases, leading to more difficulty in arousing. In other words, the disconnections between sensory and motor systems that occur during sleep, and the relative activity of one with regard to the other are reversed in these two major subdivisions of sleep, REM sleep and NREM sleep.

THE PRINCIPLES UNDERLYING MODELS

When dealing with an event that occurs in the no-man's land between the biological sciences and the psychological sciences, it is necessary to first establish our working vocabulary. We do this so that we can establish a structural framework within which to organize our information. So here, in brief, are what I will call seven organizing concepts regarding the biological foundations of behavior.

1. **The chemical messenger**. It is now established that there are literally millions if not billions of molecules that can serve as purveyors of information to and within the brain, and serve at many different levels of function to interlink the hard-wiring of the brain's nerve cells. Some of these molecules are very ordinary and others are exotic. But whether they go by the name of neurotransmitter, neuromodulator, substrate or metabolite (to name a few), they have transformed our way of thinking about the brain.

2. **The cell message receptor**. Each cell in the body has receptor sites on its surface for the purpose of receiving information, energy, and spare parts from outside itself. As a message receiver floating in the cell membrane, this doughnut-shaped protein acts like an ignition switch, activated by the various molecular "keys" encountering it. When the right molecular key fits in, the receptor activates an enzyme within the cell which then starts some process, be it growth, information exchange, or simply cellular

housekeeping functions. The cells of the brain are particularly rich with such receptors.

3. **Enzyme variability**. Enzymes are protein substances that act as catalytic agents, affecting other substances by inducing chemical changes in them while remaining relatively unchanged and reusable themselves. The discovery that certain chemicals could alter the productivity of the nerve cell's enzymes, coupled with the discovery that certain of these enzymes could be genetically "misspelled" or be otherwise improperly formed but still retain some function, has given new meaning to the biological basis for behavioral differences among individuals. A key to understanding certain human character patterns, based on alterations in the functioning of their organic underpinnings, is contained in this concept. Each of us is somewhat like a book written in a specific language. Once we decipher the language, we can read the book, but that does not give us the power to tell, without reading, what the theme of the next book is, even though it may be written in the same language. From one brain to the next, the language is the same although the molecular "spelling" and the nerve cell "sentence structure" may differ.

4. **The food–drug continuum**. Everyone who has had a high school chemistry course knows that all foods and all drugs are chemicals. At the level of the atom, all is "chemical," nothing is artificial. More specifically, many man-made molecules that have an effect on the nervous system turn out to be mimicking endogenously occurring molecules or nutrients. With the discovery of the endorphins, the so-called natural narcotic system in the brain, the stage was set for viewing all molecules as potential information-carrying candidates, whether "natural" or man-made.

5. **The evolutionary perspective**. A fundamental conceptual breakthrough has been the increasing appreciation of the evolutionary unity of the brain. Not taking away from the dignity and sovereignty of any one organism or species, brains may be more alike than different. A neuron is a neuron whether in an ant, a snail, or a human. Furthermore, even single-celled beings like bacteria employ some

of the same information-processing techniques as brain cells. With this appreciation, and with the ability to make comparative studies across species, have come clearer paths to understanding some levels of function of the human brain. The prospect that our mood- and contemplative-regulating systems are far more like those old "chemotactic" cells of molecule-seeking bacteria than we might like to admit, may seem humbling to some. But recognition of the universality of parts of the underlying machinery still does not mean that a chimp can play Mozart.

6. **The mood, activity, and cognitive cycles**. A greatly expanded awareness of the pervasive presence of chemically modulated cycles (whether hourly, daily, monthly, or seasonally) and of the role such cycles play in our daily lives—not in terms of a cult-oriented biorhythm or astrology chart, but from a scientific approach—will give us profound insight into many momentary lapses that affect us all at one time or another. Biorhythms appear to be moving from the wings of alchemy to the stage of scientific chemistry. And, in fact, the scientific study of such rhythms turns out to be much more interesting than any magical one. The fact that animals that sleep longer tend to have shorter life spans—i.e., the length of sleep in different species of animals tends to be inversely correlated with length of life—raises interesting questions regarding the purpose that sleep may serve. But whether this life-span phenomenon is in fact related to duration of sleep rather than, for example, to a higher metabolic rate in the shorter-lived slug-a-beds, remains to be established.

7. **Multiple levels of information in the brain**. The brain is like a metropolis where different compartments deal with different information content and different information media. The medium for a perception or an intellectual judgment is as different from the medium for the transmission of an emotional reaction, as a newspaper is from a television screen. Different parts of the brain are specialized in handling one medium or another, but the crossovers and interactions are becoming increasingly understood even though they are complex. And with this understanding are

coming much hard data to replace the fuzzy, impressionistic notions about body–mind interactions.

Certainly, man does not live by chemistry alone. But in a very
real sense, it is a "bottom line." And this is so, notwithstanding
modern-day societal problems regarding substance abuse. Furthermore, despite the current tendency to confuse "compulsive"
behaviors with "addictions," and the position taken by cultists of
differing stripe, whether they be pro or con "medication," for or
against the "traditional" scientific approach to questions regarding human existence, drugs and chemicals are not necessarily
"poisons." They do not affect systems purely in a negative fashion
as some health food faddists would hold; then too, all function
cannot be explained or dealt with in terms of chemicals alone, as
some scientists with rather limited vision would hold. All extremes
of these issues surrounding the search for and use of pharmacologic agents in the treatment of human disorders can be
found with vocal devotees and adherents insisting on their view
exclusively. There is a role for advocacy, but only for particular
points of view, bolstered by reproducible supporting evidence.
This is an advocacy process in which the conclusions presented are
ultimately decided for or against, based not on emotional appeal,
but on the "appeal" of verifiable fact. It is important for the public
to be informed about the range of issues, to be aware that contro-
versy does exist and easy or sure answers do not. It is likewise
important to be somewhat familiar with who the various advocates
are: cultists demanding that all "drugs" are toxins; certain public
officials holding that mental disorders are a myth and that presumed treatment is essentially a political activity; or biologists who
exhort that only medication offers a useful approach to behavioral
problems like sleep disturbances.

WHAT SLEEP MAY BE

Sleep, like blood circulation, or digestion, or respiration for
that matter, is considered by most to be a coherent, organized and
persevering system that will function more or less autonomously as
long as no qualifying factors intervene. With "sleep," in contrast to

"circulation," however, some assume that it is necessary to add the factor of "need reduction." Certainly we have all, at one time or another, experienced the subjective component which supports this assumption . . . the overwhelming feeling of an urgent requirement for immediate sleep, a feeling which seems then to be relieved by a sense of replenishment, ostensibly provided by a sound slumber.

Some theories attempting to explain the biological function, purpose, and underlying driving force of systems (such as sleep or respiration) posit an instinctive pattern of response which is evoked in a stereotyped fashion by cues in the environment. Others posit a biorhythm, coordinated with other bodily rhythms and responsive to time cues. In either case, they both assume the presence of inborn patterns of responses that have evolved to coordinate the individual to his or her environmental circumstances with the most versatility. Such theories regarding the phenomenon or system of sleep can be divided into two major categories. One could be called "appetitive" and, like sexual behaviors or animal herd migrations, would be related to functions elicited in the presence of appropriate cues. The other could be called "homeostatic" (or "need reductive," as mentioned above), like hunger or respiration in which a depletion of some critical matter is felt to trigger the attempt to redress the imbalance.

The range of conjectures regarding the function of sleep, as well as the purposes that sleeping might serve for the sleeper, has covered possibilities like the following:

1. Sleep allows restoration and recovery of mind and/or body. Although "rest" is for the body, "sleep" is for the brain and provides the occasion both for bodily rest and for increased brain protein synthesis.

2. Sleep allows this aforementioned recovery to occur by permitting the sleeper to most efficiently rest while simultaneously sampling the surrounding sleep environment for danger . . . this, by cyclical shifts into and out of lighter and then more responsive stages of sleep . . . testing the environmental waters, figuratively speaking.

3. Sleep allows respite from the continual stimulation of waking life, thereby protecting the brain from putative "burnout."

4. Sleep permits the conservation of energy either by keeping the body at rest or by a rationing imposed by the brain upon itself for specific timed periods. Here we turn to the evolutionists who see the phenomenon of sleep as a residuum, left from a previous age where it served the life-sustaining function of energy conservation. These theorists might point to sleep as they would to the intestine's appendix, or, more mundanely, to the tracks of a long-defunct municipal trolley system: the presence is still felt, but the original function that it subserved is no longer apparent. To such investigators, sleep may represent the vestige of a universal energy-conserving plan that developed for warm-blooded animals. Perhaps, they might reason, sleep was initially the behavioral component of this mechanism and, as evolution progressed, it diverged somewhat from its founding function.

5. Sleep allows cognitive and thought-processing functions to occur, or is an epiphenomenon of the grand orchestration of multiple bodily rhythms. Perhaps sleep serves different developmental functions at different times of an individual's life, or reinforces memory, or allows rehearsal and hence improvement in subsequent functioning.

As in the early stages of any science, there are many general theories regarding the purpose and role of sleep, some ingenious, some half-baked. In any case, in Chapter 2 we will have a chance to look more closely at some of these. But here it should also be mentioned that theorizing about the function of sleep has also focused on the subdivisions of REM sleep and NREM sleep.

With regard to REM sleep, some theorize that this state allows the processing of information accumulated by the individual's brain during the previous day, with the subsequent integration of some of the data into memory stores and the elimination of trivial or superfluous messages. Of course, such theories leave completely unanswered questions as to how such selections and filings are accomplished. It is of interest to note that such theoretical formulations were at the foundation of animal experiments which suggested that properties of sleep, like its stages and timing, were in part determined by the features of the immediately preceding waking experience. We will discuss more of this in Chapter 4 when we look at the reciprocal relationships that exist between sleeping life and waking experience.

An additional theory, not directly addressing questions regarding the function of sleep in general, suggests a role for REM sleep within the overall structure of sleep. This theory is developed as follows: Deep stage 4 or slow wave sleep (the deepest stage of NREM sleep) involves the marked dampening of significant portions of brain functioning. But theorists here assume that the central nervous system cannot tolerate long periods of suppressed function, any more than it can tolerate prolonged absence of oxygen. So, since part and parcel of the sleep phenomenon is the restraint of neuronal functioning, they opine that built within normal sleep cycles are periodic bouts of arousal within sleep. This REM sleep stage allows the basic sleep process to proceed while providing periodic tonic stimulation to the muffled brain, thereby allowing it to maintain its "tone." The assumption here is that the brain, if inactivated below a critical threshold for too long a time, cannot be sustained. The purpose of REM sleep therefore would either be one of "priming the pump" for action (by cyclic arousal to a subawakening threshold where sleep is still maintained but receptivity to external stimuli is enhanced and periodic sampling of the environment is possible) or one of keeping the brain alert at some minimal level of function so that the general capacity for neuronal action is sustained. It is as if the brain were a car motor, idling at a very low whisper. Every now and then you must apply your foot to the accelerator, feed the idling engine and "rev" it so that it can power movement without stalling, once the forward gears are engaged. Such a theory might go one step further and suggest that, from nature's point of view, REM sleep represents a solution to the trade-off between the necessity of sleep in order to maintain the brain's integrity and the danger to which sleep may expose the sleeping organism, either in the form of an external predator attacking the vulnerable sleeper, or as an internal loss of brain tonicity. REM sleep would let the sleeper sleep while periodically sampling the surroundings and/or recharging the recuperating brain. More of these theories will be discussed in Chapter 6.

In our exploration of sleep, we will approach the issue from both sides of the looking glass, mind and brain. These are not mutually exclusive views, but rather overlapping areas of scientific endeavor. Each of these views has been recently enriched by a wealth of exciting findings. Certainly it would be fair to state that more facts about sleep have been established in the past few years than in all earlier history. Unfortunately, however, much of this new knowledge has not found its way to the general public, and indeed little has even filtered through to the majority in the helping professions. Thus, this book will attempt to render many of these facts meaningful and, I hope, will serve as a guide to renewed self-education efforts at all levels of expertise, from the interested layman to the practicing physician. Never more than today, with rapid changes occurring within the medical sciences and within the health-care delivery systems, has it been necessary for all of us to quicken our education on topics of personal health. We shall see that the phenomenon of sleep will prove to be a very interesting example of how anyone can make sense of a diversity of new facts and understand new concepts without falling for sterile, overly facile "easy answers."

At least one-third of American adults complain of insomnia to some degree. And, with one out of eight of us resorting to sleeping pills (either prescribed or over-the-counter) in the pursuit of a restful night's sleep, it is clear that sleep is no small problem for more than 30 million people in the United States alone. "Poor sleepers" tend to be more restless during sleep and also exhibit higher pulse rates and body temperatures. These so-called poor sleepers also tend to report feelings of being awake even while objective records of their sleep activity document the fact that they are in dreamland!

When discussing what can go wrong with sleep from a clinical point of view, it is important to remember that, like Rome, each sleep disturbance can be reached via many different roads. All behavioral symptoms are multidetermined. That is, there are many different origins possible for any one behavioral phenomenon. And sleep is no exception. So, despite perhaps similar presenting symptoms, different disrupted sleep patterns and their associated pathological states can result from disruption in the organic function of brain tissue, environmental changes, behavioral stress and so forth—and, as such, should not be treated as a unitary phenomenon. For the same apparent condition can reflect different underlying states in different individuals, or in the same individual at different times. In this regard, it should also be noted that sleep disorders can therefore tell us something about specific individuals, and that the diagnostic investigation of sleep patterns can provide us with useful information about other pathological states such as depression, alcoholism, and certain medical diseases.

After reviewing basic theoretical and conceptual information on the phenomenon of sleep, and after discussing the possible functions of sleep from the points of view of protection, restoration, growth, memory consolidation, and adaptation to the sleeper's ecological niche, the range of varied sleep patterns, from healthy to unhealthy, will be reviewed. Then we will turn to the influence of external substances on the regulation of sleeping and waking.

Beginning with the first physicians (in effect, cooks dealing with natural herbs), all the way to modern-day neurochemists and clinical researchers, man has sought to create specific potions and concoctions in an attempt to affect mood states and the sleep–wake cycle. From ancient Greek and Aztec practices through the practices of early modern medicine, the search has proceeded for sleep-enhancing drugs, for a balm of sleep. Nowadays, with an increasingly sophisticated consumer population, it is important to note some of the underlying attitudes toward the use of medication which various advocacy groups espouse. No longer caught up in primitive animistic superstition like the Druids who would burn their captives in wicker cages while they would "get in touch with the infinite," modern man has not yet fully embraced the power of the scientific method. He still seeks magical solutions to some of the existential qualities, if not problems, of life. Whether "hippies" in the drug culture of the 60s, "yuppies" in the "me" generation of the 80s, or the emerging "New-Agers" of the 90s, movements have always been afoot that have attempted to modify aspects of the human condition or at least to try to soothe the confrontations with them. Inevitably, with such movements, questions are raised about what phenomena are unavoidable and part of being human, and what phenomena are the result of inner failures to live up to "potential." Likewise inevitably, questions will be raised as to what is an "illness" and what needs to be "cured." "Reality" can then be considered as a mere social construct, relative only to other reference points around the person. Knowledge itself becomes merely a construct as well, rather than a revelation of underlying fixed truths.

Concerning doctrinaire struggles between biological psychiatrists and psychoanalysts, between medical practitioners and consumer advocate groups, between medical researchers and those who would invoke human rights or religious authority as a rationale for stopping selected research activities . . . yes, even between evolutionary theorists and the "creationists" . . . one cannot help but be reminded of the fable of the elephant and the blind men, in which multiple observers from multiple perspectives describe the same phenomenon differently. With regard to the brain and the behavioral sciences, each "blind man," be he medical researcher, psychological theorist, poet, or theologian, is correct but limited in his interpretation of the "elephant," sleep. And for each of these "blind men" humility would be a welcome trait. For with the on-rushing, exponentially increasing volume of new information regarding brain function swirling around us, much of the way we view human activity is bound to change. Just as Copernicus, Darwin, and then Freud led us to a more humble perspective of our role in the cosmos and on our planet, so these new discoveries will modify our perspective of human will and spirit: our planet is "only" one of many around an ordinary star in an ordinary galaxy; we are "only" a primate among other primates; our conscious is not only contending with the obvious but with a far larger arena, our unconscious. Those of us who took excessive pride in the autonomy of our brains are going to have to reconcile themselves with the fact that we function at the behest of ancestral appetites known even to the lowly bacterium. And in this era of burgeoning information, and ironically as a consequence of increasing questioning, nothing will turn off the continued progress toward knowledge faster than the repeated tendency of cultists to take one observation in isolation and surround it with pseudoscientific mumbo jumbo, and perhaps a curious brand of anti-intellectualism—even though, as most students of history know, many scientific disciplines arose from such prescientific pursuits as alchemy and astrology.

THE PURPOSE OF AN INTERDISCIPLINARY APPROACH

Sleep behavior among human beings appears to depend upon multiple factors which do not always act with the same intensity or in the same pattern. Sleep is not only an essential and vital life process, it is also a particularly informative instance of behavior because it makes details from biochemical, physiological, behavioral and sociological research increasingly available. Each of these areas deals with part of the total phenomenon of sleep. Each area has its own metaphor, but each covers only part of the problem, largely taking the other aspects for granted (as we will see when we examine the world of dreams). To begin to understand the whole, however, requires first, that the various metaphors be put together as pieces in a puzzle, and second, that they be made to map in some way on each other so that metaphors in parallel end up enriching, rather than competing with, each other.

These are some of the objectives of this book, and where issues of self-assessment and self-help are discussed, these objectives come into particular focus. For, although there is a biological basis to behavior, behavior such as sleep is not controlled exclusively by biological factors. As will become more apparent, none of the theoretical or research models adequately describes the whole sleep cycle, though each may account for part of it. Questions must be related to how the appropriate physiological and biochemical processes map onto behavioral patterns. Such questions, however, are easily asked but not so easily answered.

When we address sleep problems, we are talking about particular physiological events (in the sleep cycle) which begin with relatively unambiguous meaning, that over time become embedded in the individual's experience in different ways. To approach self-help within this context of the sleep experience requires a scientific mode of thinking. Each person has to develop a sense of civilized self-awareness of his or her structure and function so that he or she becomes literate in the understanding of certain biological and psychological issues. As practical consequences of this awareness, the individual will begin to develop the ability to make enlightened distinctions between problems and nonproblems; he or she will know when to seek professional help, serving as an "assistant diagnostician" in the process; and he or she can address other areas of his or her life that may directly influence the sleep—wake cycle . . . areas such as nutrition, exercise, lifestyle, and general physical and psychological health.

The connection between general health and mind has been wisely noted for centuries. However, the sense of something vague and purely spiritual has often left this area of investigation in the hands of philosophers. Frequently, medical men will pay lip service to this concept, but in practice will hand out tranquilizers to those patients in whom nothing "organic" can be found. Most likely what is in fact happening is that they have been looking for the lesion, in these "functional" illnesses, in the wrong place. Furthermore, in conditions as serious as hypertension, myocardial infarction, and even cancer, the most significant "lesion" may be in the brain. And it is with the study of sleep that we have really begun to appreciate the function of this organ, the brain, in the development and maintenance of psychosomatic and neurosomatic phenomena.

As more has been learned about the "spelling" of those special proteins called enzymes, it has been recognized that minor hereditary differences in the building block components of the enzyme (that is, in its amino acids) can modify its function without totally disabling it. Increasingly, it is these minor structural modifications of these essential cogs in the basic machinery of the cell, body, and brain, that are proving to be the key to the so-called "functional" illnesses.

We are beginning to appreciate subtle variations in certain neuron populations, besides variations in enzymes which occur in all but identical twins (and possibly in some of them as well). Out of the over 100 billion neurons in the human brain, about 10,000 manufacture an alerting chemical called noradrenalin. A close cousin of this, dopamine, is made in perhaps 50,000 cells. If a sizable portion of this relatively small number of cells is destroyed, the individual becomes comatose (as, for example, in sleeping sickness). Less drastic alterations of this cell population may affect aspects of the human personality along its entire spectrum, resulting in changes in processes running the continuum from those considered "physiological" to those considered "temperamental." As we learn more and more, and as the brain and its functioning "mind" yields more to penetrating inquiry and thereby becomes less of a mysterious black box, we come closer to doing away with the twin tragedies of the doctor's patient with his "brainless body" and the psychiatrist's patient with his "brainless mind." The study of sleep is just that sort of fabled "elephant" spoken of before. It is now being looked at, simultaneously, from multiple perspectives. And it is in the neurosciences that we provide the occasion for the interdisciplinary meeting of the "blind men" which we shall now attend.

Chapter 2

The ABCs of Catching Zs—
Normal Sleep, What It Is
From Rest to Slumber
to Hibernation

"Honey, go to sleep now," says the Mommy. "Why do I have to?!" the child demands and, with that response, asks a questions that goes far beyond the dynamics of a familiar moment in the bedtime struggle. Why do we "have to" go to sleep? What is this mysterious one-third of our lives we call sleep, and what are its normal patterns? How do these change over an individual's lifetime? What do we know about the range of healthy variation in sleep patterns as a person grows and ages? And, of course, "why?" Why do we sleep at all . . . what possible functions does sleep serve?

To attempt to answer these questions (questions which, incidentally, represent only the tip of the iceberg of inquiries that might be made about sleep), we must first be in possession of a consistently valid and reliable definition of the phenomenon of "sleep." The fact that we so suddenly are carried off in the arms of Morpheus once we fall into sleep, may suggest a galvanic process in which a switch is thrown, suddenly carrying us into new territories, neurologically and psychologically speaking. Once we can define what sleep is, then, perhaps, we will be able to more clearly delineate and describe some of these qualities.

So, first, we must be able to talk to each other in a meaningful way so that when I say "sleep," or "awake" . . . or state of "vigilance" or "torpor" for that matter, you will know to what phenomenon, characterized by what events, I am referring. To do this, a sound and robust definition of "sleep", which will allow us to talk to each other about the state, is necessary.

TECHNIQUES FOR EXPLORING SLEEP

To many, it may seem that the definition of sleep is self-evident. Well it is not, and, in the not too distant past, it was even less so. Before the advent of techniques for monitoring the electrophysiological activity of brain cells, sleep was defined by behavioral actions considered to be characteristic of a sleeping creature. Thus, a beast was said to be asleep if it was relatively immobile, relatively unresponsive to external disturbances, and had assumed a typical "sleeping" posture. This circular definition, that an animal was sleeping if it acted as if it were sleeping, was applied to all mammals and allowed at least for the recognition of several salient features of the sleeping state. One of these features was the presence of a protective "stimulus-barrier," a shield that prevented external excitement from arousing the sleeper, yet could be reversed in the face of survival demands from overwhelming or imperative environmental alerts. Several additional characteristics that were used to further define sleep included descriptive variables such as the length of the sleeping episode and the timing of its occurrence within the 24-hour day.

With the advent of electroencephalogram (EEG) technology, electrical patterns of brain cell activity could be detected, recorded and thereby compared with contemporaneously occurring behavioral events of the organism possessing those brain cells. When the first EEG's of the brain's electrical activity were recorded in 1929, the stage was set for a later moment in 1937 when it was recognized that sleep was not just a simple, homogeneous steady state, nor a random, undisciplined occurrence. Rather, sleep was a process divided into a complex series of stages. Sixteen years later, the cyclic nature of these stages began to be appreciated. Then the close correspondence between the characteristics of sleep–wake behavior patterns and the motifs of sleep–wake brain cell electrical activity could be noted. Thus a new tool led to the development of a new dimension in the definition and delineation of the phenomenon of sleep, and the door was opened to an avalanche of studies aimed at exploring factors that might initiate, maintain, or disrupt the sleep event.

Early observers noted that we fall asleep mostly by lapsing first into a deep sleep stage which is associated with a considerable amount of hormonal activity—just to name a few of the neuroendocrine agents mobilized during this stage of sleep: melatonin, cortisol, growth hormone, and thyrotropin. Additional observations were made regarding the alteration in other bodily processes during sleep as the initial deep stage 4 sleep (or slow wave, as it is sometimes called, with its characteristic "slow," discursive wave forms on EEG tracings), alternates with the dreamy REM stage of sleep, with its characteristic rapid eye movements. From the observations of the behavioral and physiological correlates of the sleep stages developed many theories regarding the purpose of sleep. These ranged from the "sentinel hypothesis" (suggesting that the purpose of shifts among different depths of sleep was to allow both for rest and yet periodic near-arousal, just in case danger was near and flight was indicated), to the REM state as a dream factory; from theories of tonic brain stimulation, bodily repair, and growth, to hypotheses about memory consolidation.

So, observations were made, initial questions posed, and preliminary theoretical constructs proposed. How, then, were the next phase of questions to be approached? Well, a procedure, familiar to other fields of medical research, was entertained. Here, an organ is removed, or its function is interfered with and the investigator sees what happens, or, rather, in this case, what doesn't happen. This represents a rather crude but often effective way of determining a system's function. Suppose, for instance, you have just bought a magnificent old Victorian mansion— admittedly a "handyman's special"—but a magnificent old beauty, with great filigreed detail, massive sweeping porches overlooking a grand rolling lawn, lots of cozy nooks and crannies . . . and an electrical system that is a tangled, jumbled, defunct mess. You must now dissect the electrical pathways, rewire and consolidate the function of the basement electrical command center by figuring out what's connected to what, and what is functioning. Well, the way to get clues about the function of your electrical system is to systematically "pull the plug" on subsections of the system and see then what no longer works. So, step by step you disconnect one fuse after another, checking the outlets affected after each disruption.

In a somewhat similar fashion, much of the early basic biological search for an understanding of the purpose and function of a biological process or organ is characterized by attempts to remove it, turn it off, or hold it in abeyance, and then see what happens. It was hoped that from similar pokings, testings, proddings, and explorings, the answer to questions regarding the functional purposes and consequences of sleep might follow.

Now with the advent of even newer technologies it is felt that sleep researchers will be able to make the transition from purely psychological levels of inquiry to levels of study which encompass the neuroanatomical and neurophysiological foundations of the behavioral state as well. Images of areas deep within the brain of the living subject can now be captured with the use of magnetic resonance imaging (MRI) and computer assisted tomography (CAT) techniques. The CAT scan is able to provide serial X-ray pictures of the brain, for instance, like slices through a loaf of bread, and then to reconstruct a three-dimensional representation of structures deep within that "loaf." MRI also gives information about structures within bodily organs, in this case, by sensing the magnetic fields created by the very atomic components of these different structures and then constructing a pictorial map from them. In fact, from studies using this technique in humans, it has been found that changes in structural parts of specific brain areas may be associated with forms of depression and schizophrenia. The neuronal activity of discrete structures within the brain can be detected and monitored using regional blood-flow (RBF) studies. And even those most microscopic and chemical of processes, the metabolic sequences within individual cells, can now be scrutinized in the living individual with advanced imaging techniques called positron-emission tomography (PET) or single photon-emission tomography. Like a satellite circling the earth and sensing differences in heat and light which are then translated into a pictorial representation of differential population densities,

PET creates an image by transducing the minute and subtle bits of metabolic information generated at a submicroscopic level into a macroscopic picture of a functioning organ.

THE SCOPE OF SLEEP ACROSS SPECIES

Sleep, as opposed to rest or mere inactivity, is, it would seem, a relatively new phenomenon in the history of life on earth. Although we can still only employ informed speculation as to its ultimate function in our lives, it is interesting to look at some of the data from seemingly unconnected "basic" scientific research. Fields as far apart as biochemistry and astrophysics have tidbits to contribute to this puzzle. For example, investigations of the remains of an ancient form of the shellfish, the chambered nautilus, appear to show a correlation between its growth and the shorter lunar month that prevailed at an earlier epoch in the earth's history. We have long been able to correlate growth rings on trees, with one ring per annual growing season. Work with the modern chambered nautilus has suggested that the creature creates one section of shell per lunar month, perhaps as a result of tidal alterations affected by the moon's period of orbit around the earth. This creature has inhabited the planet for quite some time so that fossils of its direct and unmistakable ancestors are available for study. But when examined, the monthly chambers of these forefathers from hundreds of millions of years ago seemed foreshortened, as if the growing cycle was shorter. It soon became apparent that the presumed shorter growth cycle of the ancient shellfish correlated rather well with the shorter orbit time of the moon around the earth. Those who study lunar mechanics have been able to estimate quite accurately, with the aid of inventions such as laser rangefinders, how much the moon is currently receding from the earth each year. In short, when the chambered nautilus was a boy, the moon was much closer to the earth and revolved around it much faster, the tides came and went at a faster pace, and the creature had to build its shell sections in a shorter time frame.

There may be those of you now murmuring "What, for Pete's sake, does this have to do with the human condition?!" Well, this shellfish is telling us something about biological clocks, a subject that most certainly bears on the human condition in sickness and health, and is essential to our understanding of the sleep–wake cycle. It even relates to those murmurers in the audience suffering from jet lag as they read this book on their transoceanic flight. This is but one example of a biological clock, and though it is the most ancient yet discovered, it did not surface until recently.

Many people, at one time or another, have had to solve a puzzle involving connecting points with a pencil in a drawing without taking the pencil off the paper. They were stumped until they ventured outside the confines of the drawing. This classic lesson in the need to change perspective crops up again and again in the history of all human endeavor and particularly in scientific problem-solving. For us to understand sleep, we must know its history. The study of evolution is rather like taking that pencil outside the confines of the puzzle drawing. For it is through the study of other life forms that we can begin to differentiate between the characteristics of sleep as compared to mere inactivity.

Thanks to our ability to study the brains of other animals more directly, we have, for openers, established that there are sleep centers in the brain. Through the discipline of comparative neuroanatomy and neurophysiology, we have traced these centers back in evolutionary time to an epoch when the brain lacked these.

Virtually all warm-blooded animals (mammals and birds) do sleep. This has been established by documenting the close correspondence between the EEG electrical patterns reflective of brain cell sleep activity and the overtly observable behaviors we have come to recognize as representing the sleep state in the animals studied. Although it is recognized that such electrographic changes can at times be recorded in animals in states other than sleep, it is the fact that these changes (both electrographic and behavioral) often occur together that provides us with this working definition of the sleeping state. Predators, like the big cats, are good sleepers, whereas animals subject to significant predation tend not to be. Despite knowing this, however, we should not give in to the tendency to look for parallel human indicators in this regard in an attempt to classify the more predatory personality types amongst us from the total amount of sleep characteristically taken!

With regard to sleep duration in humans, infants spend 50 percent of their time in sleep while adults spend a third of their day and the elderly, about 6 hours a day. There are documented cases of a few individuals who get by with only a few hours of sleep each night, although maybe they catch several evanescent, mini-naps during the day. Normal sleep periods can range from the reported 5 hours per night for Napoleon, to the more than 9 hours per night for Einstein. It is difficult for anyone to maintain a vigil beyond four days of sleep deprivation. With chronic, but slightly less extreme deprivation, the development of a dementia-like condition (with memory disturbances and impaired thinking and judgment) has been noted. Such observations regarding consistent and expectable patterns of sleep and of response to sleep loss, further support our intuitive appreciation of the importance, as yet unspecified, of sleep for human beings.

As we travel back in evolutionary time along the phylogenetic scale to vertebrates such as reptiles, amphibians, and fish, and then even further "back" to the invertebrate insects, we run into a state characterized by behavioral inactivity coupled with a responsiveness to external stimuli rather than a stimulus insensitivity. This is a halfway nonsleep, drowsy state with normal, waking level thresholds to environmental stimulation. It is not yet clear to what extent such a state represents the precursor of the sleeping state found in birds and mammals. Questions regarding sleep in fish and the varieties of sleep-like phenomena in different aquatic mammals are just a few of the fascinating points remaining to be clarified to fill in our descriptive spectrum of sleep across the species. For instance, killer whales or bottle-nosed porpoises have been demonstrated to sleep while swimming. Like great airships, put on "hold," they quietly circle in stereotypic counterclockwise patterns, suspended in their liquid medium until awakened by some inner "control tower" that announces the end of "hanging" time. Or consider the observation that dolphins apparently sleep, one side of the brain at a time. They seem to alternate between left and right hemispheres with no apparent REM sleep at all. It would seem to be difficult to do all that neurological juggling . . . and to dream as well!

It is with the reptiles that we first see the suggestion of the sleep-like state characteristic of birds and mammals, rather than the omnipresent "resting" of amphibians, fish, and invertebrates. Answers to questions regarding the "sleep" of creatures from the languorous alligator to the apparently impassive lizard, to the inert chameleon, and the unaroused snake are not yet available. Whether or not this state of repose is the same for all reptiles and whether or not it represents an evolutionary transition point from the behavioral stillness of fish to fully developed sleep, will have to await further study.

Perhaps the larger point in our observations here is that, regardless of the details of the process observed, as we trace it through the interlocking species to reveal a historical reflection of evolution known as phylogeny, an enormous number of organisms take time out from their daily rounds to assume an entirely different behavioral state. This state is characterized by certain expected and stereotypical behaviors often carried out in specific environmental niches and distinguished by a reversible state of decreased behavioral responsiveness and arousal. It seems that most multicellular animals, even as far down the evolutionary ladder as the insect, kick off their shoes and relax. The range of rest times is broad: the cockroach can rest for 14 hours in the crack of a kitchen floorboard, while the sand piper sleeps only for 3 hours, as do the horse and the elephant. Regardless of whether we look at the gorilla or the woodchuck, each of which sleeps away 80 to 90 percent of his life, and regardless of how the total sleep time may be distributed during the 24-hour cycle, they all do it. Whether under a leaf, in a cave, quietly circling in the night ocean, or high above the midnight crowd in a cramped studio apartment, we all "crash." Certain variations can be observed in the patterns of sleep, as such factors as seasonal changes (for instance in cold-blooded animals), age (with length of sleep decreasing in humans as age progresses), or nutritional requirements affect the profile. But we all sleep. Or do we? As can well be imagined, it is difficult to be completely sure that there is no bird or mammal that does not sleep, although there is the assumption that the albatross, in its pelagic journeys, sleeps very little. This oceanic voyager may be like the marathon dancers of the 30s and 40s who, totally exhausted and propping each other up, would catch a wink or two while still moving.

THOUGHTS ON EVOLUTION AND THE PURPOSE OF SLEEP

But if we all sleep, why do we do so? What is the purpose of this apparent rest period? And what can we know about the purpose of sleep in humans, specifically? The surgical removal of an organ may reveal its functional significance, which had not yet been identified before. Some investigators feel that in the same manner, sleep "deprivation" might elucidate the purpose and function of sleep if careful attention were paid to the consequences of such interventions in experimental subjects. An additional research tactic taken by some early researchers involved the close observation of phenomena that might be present when an individual is forcibly awakened at different times of the night, from different stages of sleep. The reasoning was that perhaps the transition between different stages of sleep and waking states, and the effect of this forced transition on subsequent mental performance, might reflect something of the nature of the patterns of brain activity and the shifts that occur among them during different stages of the sleep–activity cycle.

The overall conclusion from animal studies is that total sleep deprivation is fatal and that partial sleep deprivation (for instance, the selective deprivation of just REM sleep) is likewise fatal, but with a more delayed effect. Specifically, early studies involving animals suggested that sleep deprivation leads to significant disruption in energy metabolism and body temperature regulation, and to the deterioration of body structures that can ultimately be lethal. However, no evidence has yet been found to confirm that brain function is outrightly disabled. Of course, we cannot interview animals. For ethical as well as volitional reasons, human studies of sleep deprivation cannot be carried out to such an extreme that metabolic and energetic results become as potentially dire as in the animal studies. But, although only shorter periods of sleep deprivation can be imposed on human subjects as compared with their animal counterparts, humans can be talked to, reassured, and monitored more closely so that researchers have the opportunity to assess the functional psychological consequences of sleep loss and thereby catch a glimpse, perhaps of the significance, of the entire phenomenon.

In this regard, selective REM sleep deprivation studies involving humans have suggested that brain activity is affected by even relatively small amounts of such loss, including changes in learning and memory, the relief of depression, and the heightening of fantasies in subjects whose imaginative activity had previously been rather impoverished.

Although there has been a temptation for many investigators to see in sleep an adaptive or recuperative role for the body as a whole, a look at differences in bodily functions during sleep and during waking life suggests that sleep primarily affects the brain and not other organs. Subtly interwoven energic functions notwithstanding, the rest of the body (other than the brain) does not seem to go into any state specific to sleep that is functionally distinctive from other states of activity. For instance, the extent of muscle readiness for action (as measured by studies of oxygen consumption) is reduced minimally during sleep. But the brain operates significantly differently when asleep and, depending on the stage of the sleep cycle, may range from a state of quiet but prepared calm to one of sensory disengagement and reduced responsiveness to external stimuli.

The previously mentioned tendency for some to assume a reparative or restitutive and maintenance function for sleep, was supported by evidence suggesting an increased secretion of the anabolic agent growth hormone (GH) into the bloodstream during stages of deep, slow wave sleep. Much like the nighttime road crews repairing the scars of heavy daytime traffic, sleep was viewed as the mender of the Shakespearean "ravelled sleave." Just one further step is required to extend this restorative function reasoning to the mental work of the brain, and to propose that sleep allows the sorting, indexing and perhaps storing or discarding of the mental accumulations of the day's activities. Support for this latter supposition has been marshalled from studies reporting the falloff in attention and memory after bouts of sleep deprivation, and from those postulating improvement in mental efficiency with increased amounts of slow wave sleep. But initially, it was from studies of the effects of both exercise and sleep deprivation that the hypothesis regarding the restorative function of sleep evolved. The observation specifically was that both the percentage of slow wave sleep and the blood level of GH were significantly raised at night, following marked physical exertion. These findings, coupled with the subjective reports of those who had exercised vigorously were taken to support the contention that sleep is an important restorer following physical wear and tear.

In seeming contradiction to what was noted before, researchers observed shifts in bodily functions which occurred during sleep. These included increased protein manufacture by cells as well as increased cellular division (mitosis), with the implication that cellular growth was stimulated during sleep, an observation with potential significance for the timing of cancer chemotherapy. Additionally, it was noted that the secretion of GH was increased and that of adrenal corticosteroids was decreased during sleep. GH is a hormone secreted by the brain's pituitary gland, and is involved with the preferential metabolism of fats and with the concomitant sparing of protein from the metabolic furnaces during fasting. It is assumed, but not proven, to be an agent important for tissue growth. From these observations, many reached the conclusion that sleep provided an opportunity for repair and recovery from the trials of the previous day's activities.

However, on closer examination of these phenomena which are presumed to be evidence in support of the bodily restitution-function theory of sleep, it becomes clear that sleep is the **occasion** for inactivity, and as such may only indirectly account for the metabolic and physiologic changes observed in the muscles, glands and other organs during sleep. In fact, these changes may occur irrespective of the brain's "sleeping" state, and may be present when the body is in repose, whether or not the brain is sleeping.

To determine whether sleep helps to conserve brain energy as opposed to being the occasion for total body rest (and, therefore, total body energy conservation), we would have to know whether there is a significant decrease in brain energy utilization during sleep. Such information is not yet available. So, studies which report the destruction of body tissue in animals subjected to sleep deprivation, even in the face of increased food consumption, or studies which suggest that wound healing is speeded up during sleep, still do not answer the question as to whether these effects are directly related to sleep, or are the concomitants of sleep-enforced "rest." Furthermore, it was discovered that the availability of amino acid building blocks harvested from that dinner meal's digestion, several hours before sleep, is the critical influence on steroid hormone production and subsequent protein synthesis—not the sleep state itself. Actually, later on in sleep, after the bulk of previously ingested food is digested, and its by-products absorbed and metabolized, the body cells experience a normal, cyclical breakdown in some of the protein stores as sleep progresses and turns into a limited fast . . . a fast that remains until broken by the first meal of the next day. So it may be that sleep itself is not the direct cause of body restitution and cell growth but only one of the particular occasions during which such restorative processes occur.

As with many other bodily functions in humans, even the very rhythm of cellular division is orchestrated by an internal circadian maestro. Here, peaks in this tissue-growth activity (from liver and intestinal cells, to skin and nails) occur at night, and here too this phenomenon seems to be more a function of inactivity than of the sleep state itself. For example, intermediating factors such as amount of preceding physical exercise, feeding, and the concomitant levels of steroid hormones and adrenalin in the blood are important effectors of the activity of the cellular division processes. It just so happens that most often, during sleep, there occurs a confluens of these factors, in optimal proportions, that leads to an increase in mitotic activity.

What about other speculations regarding the function of sleep? To proceed, it is first important to note that early life forms contain simplified physiological and behavioral "maps" that can be used as guides to understanding the vastly more complex nature of our own nervous systems and our attendant behavior. To anyone not acquainted with studies of the brains of various species it may be startling to realize how marked the degree of continuity is in the microscopic structure of brains in organisms as remote in origin from each other as sharks, bumblebees and human beings. The basic functioning unit of all nervous systems, even those one would not dignify with the appellation "brain," is the nerve cell or neuron. The neuron can be recognized by the neurobiologist in various species almost as easily as a mechanic might recognize an old spark plug. Although the neuron does come in hundreds of sizes and shapes (some three hundred have been identified in humans), its basic mechanism has remained unchanged from the jellyfish to the homo sapiens.

And the continuities among species go beyond just structural considerations to similarities in basic physiological processes as well. Whether or not fish "sleep" while swimming (as noted before in aquatic mammals such as porpoises and killer whales), all creatures so far studied exhibit periodic cycles of activity and inactivity, and in almost all animals studied, these cycles are keyed in some way to light–dark photoperiodicity. And whether porpoise or shark, eagle or aardvark, all animals have similar basic neurological components that allow them to take their place in the study of the phenomenon of sleep, even as it might relate to humans.

Because of this tendency toward the conservation of life technology, all manner of living things contain similar nuts and bolts. Even plants, which have no nervous systems, but do have similar chemical sensor and messenger or hormone systems, share many chemical subunits with us. Thus no work on any life form, however seemingly remote from us, can be dismissed out of hand as irrelevant. In fact, because some forms, such as aplysia and squid, have more accessible nervous systems, they make excellent candidates for basic neuron research.

Most of us know that all higher life forms on earth today use DNA as the genetic blueprint material for passing on hereditary information, but few of us may be aware that all nervous systems show a strong family resemblance as well. For example, the drug diazepam (Valium®) is able to attach itself to the neurons of all manner of land- and air-dwelling creatures and all bony fishes in the sea because the neurons of these animals whether bird, beast, or denizen of the deep, have biochemical structures, called receptors, that are similar. One has to go all the way back to the shark, a fellow of very primitive lineage, before Valium® becomes irrelevant. With him, however, we can still use morphine as a brainstem tonic, and morphine works way past his primitive relatives until we reach creatures without a backbone, like the octopus. From here back to single-celled creatures, we can often get an effect with lecithin or other substances that yield acetylcholine, which in multicelled animals serves as a neurotransmitter, part of the communication system between neurons. But even in single-celled organisms, creatures with no neurons, this future neurotransmitter is present and functions in some role inside that cell, awaiting its big turn on life's evolutionary stage.

We can liken a neuron to a motor that can be run on a number of different fuels and linked with other motors to form a very complex instrument. It would appear that evolutionary early brains had fewer motors with a restricted range of fuels. As time progressed, however, a new fuel was discovered and added to the repertory, larger motor arrays were added, and new array combinations were devised. Those who have followed the more recent and rapid evolution of computer circuit design will be struck by the parallel. Today, more than three hundred different types of "motors" exist in the human brain and there are a good two dozen candidates for "fuel." It should be noted, though, that no new types of "fuel" have been discovered since the shark, and the evolution of brains in warm-blooded creatures appears to be strictly one of different arrays with different quantitative investments depending on need. The whale and the bat invest a lot of neurons in sonar and radar, respectively. We humans use the same model "motors and fuel" to process visual and auditory information of a more familiar type. Probably the basic "motor" used in the highest of human brain functions, speech (and related symbolic and abstracting processes), is no different from the neurons used by the whale and the bat for correlating sensory data from various sources in the environment.

The happy fact that the evolutionary process did conserve such an astounding percentage of its technological tricks allows scientists to draw a very large number of conclusions about probable human brain function from animal brain studies. Unfortunately, however, when it comes to the brain, scientists are in somewhat the same position that Galileo was in regarding his views of the solar system. One never fails to hear the caveat that animal research cannot be applied too directly to humans, especially when it deals with brain or mind issues. While it is certainly true the rats are not humans, and that the vast increase in brain size and pattern redesign in the human brain would make unwise any automatic translation of rat brain findings to humans, it is equally unwise to have a knee-jerk reaction of skepticism to any recent animal brain finding as applied to people. In such reactions one may suspect a political motive, or perhaps a lingering hankering for the kind of archaic vitalism that refused to investigate how nonliving chemical structures could evolve into living forms, but contented itself with arguing that such evolution was basically impossible without supernatural help. The sin of hubris rests more with those who would keep man supernaturally apart from the rest of life, than with those who would investigate the natural connections.

BRAIN FUNCTION AND SLEEP FUNCTION

Whenever we look at major physiological functions of the living organism, functions such as circulation, respiration, digestion and so forth, we assume the existence of an overriding organizational structure for each of these systems . . . a structure with multiple internal "bureaucratic" hierarchies. For instance, with the life-sustaining function of respiration, we tie together the following reactions and systems: chemical reactions at the cellular level (functioning as monitors of oxygen need), with exchange reactions at the lung surface intervening between life-giving air and transportation systems in the bloodstream, with signal systems within the muscles of the chest wall regulating the excursive movements during the act of breathing, with coordinating centers all the way up in the brain (which are sensitive to reports from all its outlying branches, and which are in basic control of the entire process regardless of the state of consciousness of the respiring individual). If such a structure is thought to be so for a function such as respiration, why not for sleep? It is precisely such reasoning that has led some to postulate the existence of an organizing structure arching over the various phases of the sleep–wake cycle and perhaps even including other levels of brain activity normally thought of as pathological and not included within the scope of a sleep–wake continuum. These latter would include conditions loosely called "epilepsy," "torpor," or "coma," which range along the continuum from consciousness to unconsciousness. They are different from phenomena known as "hypnotic" or "dissociative," which run along another continuum of brain activity, that of attention.

Let us view the brain, and its behavioral counterparts, as comprising different departments, as if in a large retail department store. In this comparison, each department may be seen as having its own activity schedule which must be coordinated with those of its counterpart departments. Each is governed in its activity by an executive body, and each of these administrative bodies is answerable to and regulated by an overriding agency, the central financial officer ("CFO"). This CFO allots different resources at different times, orchestrating a shifting pattern of needs, demands, and responses. So, too, with the brain we may speculate that there exists an overriding executive agency, regulating and coordinating the various brain activity "departments" and orchestrating the varying levels of activity or preparedness required while simultaneously monitoring energy expenditures and conserving resource inventories. But here, as in business life itself, the executive agency still has to answer to an even higher authority commanded by the insistent, and at times preemptory, demands of ages-old biological clocks.

Two European scientists, one a German by the name of Vieth (1986) and the other a Swiss named Koella (1986), have proposed a term for just such an executive agency with regard to sleep. They call it the bureau-for-the-regulation-of-varying-states-of-vigilance. "Vigilance," here, represents a concept of neurological and/or psychological alertness and is taken to reflect a changing state of excitation, or readiness for response, on a basic functional level, be it neuronal or psychological.

But how do we translate this proposal regarding a vigilance function to an understanding about the possible purpose of sleep? Intuitively, if in no other way, we recognize the purpose of wakefulness. It seems to be a prerequisite for getting things done! Also, empirically, we experience the effect of sleep. We feel rested and refreshed afterwards, under most circumstances. It is here that some thoughts about epilepsy, previously mentioned as a condition not ordinarily thought to lie along the sleep and wakefulness continuum, may add to our understanding regarding the function of sleep. What follows is a model of brain activity that involves coordinated but shifting levels of activity of groups of neurons which, when synchronized by some hypothetical "executive function," provide the neurophysiological basis for behavioral activity cycles. It is this system of changing but interdigitating and, at times, synchronized, neuronal activities that has been dubbed "vigilance" by Koella and Vieth.

Epileptic seizures are a form of brain cell excitement or activity and, as such, can be considered to be disorders subsumed under the rubric of what we are calling "vigilance." It is interesting to note that the seemingly chaotic state of uncontrolled brain cell electrical activity, known as a seizure, can be triggered by any one of a number of stimulus inputs to the susceptible brain. In predisposed or susceptible individuals, such stimuli run the gamut from excessive "stress" to physical over-exertion, from sleep deprivation to the transition from NREM sleep to REM sleep, from intense emotional reactions to strobe lights or music. Here, the level of receptivity or responsiveness to the provoking stimulus suggested to several researchers the existence of an overriding mechanism regulating (or in this case, "dysregulating") the level of "vigilance." This has led to the attempt to inhibit the occurrence of certain forms of epileptic seizure (pyknolepsy and the psychomotor seizures) in those suffering from the episodic disorder by encouraging the patient to increase his or her focus of concentration, interest, or distraction—that is, to increase the level of vigilance within brain systems governing alertness. This shift along the alertness continuum does in fact seem to exert strong inhibitory effects on seizures. The network of interacting neuronal cells that form the basis for an individual's moment-to-moment functioning is, it would seem, intimately related to levels of arousal; changing levels of vigilance, as occurs with changes in the sleep–wake cycle, will change the degree of synchronization in neuronal function, as occurs in epilepsy.

It is here then, in the presence of a hypothesized regulatory mechanism controlling the levels of activation or preparedness for action, that some researchers explore their theories regarding the purpose of sleep and ask whether sleep and wakefulness differ from each other in terms of actual functions present. Or, rather, whether they differ only in levels of activity and responsiveness to stimuli presented to a common set of functional systems which happen to have quantitative, not qualitative, differences in function. In other words, is one state, either sleep or arousal, a "permissive" condition that allows other events to occur (like snoring or dreaming on the one hand, or writing and eating on the other), without which substantially different functions, rather than just differences in amount of the same functions, will occur? Furthermore, is the sleeping brain like the automobile with its ignition disconnected and its engine essentially unusable; or, is it more like a revving car engine, the clutch not yet engaged, still retaining the potential for movement? Such theorizing has led investigators from the question "Why sleep at all?" to more specific hypothesizing regarding the possible purpose of the two major subdivisions sleep, REM sleep and NREM sleep.

In an effort to explore some of the background issues surrounding the search for the purpose of sleep, we must range over a huge span of time. As we do, the appearance of the phenomenon of sleep seems more and more to represent a sign of a fundamental change in the way the brain operated. If we were to arrange a series of momentous evolutionary landmarks, the origin of life itself would be at one end and the beginning of human speech might be at the other. In between would be a few unquestionable moments crucial to the progress toward intelligent life. Certainly, the rise of multicellular life (or creatures) was a momentous occasion that did not occur until life had already covered 80 percent of its present time span on this planet. Next would have to be the invention of the brain itself, with its concomitant eyes, ears, limbs, etc. After that, sleep may be the only evolutionary advance worth mentioning in such illustrious company.

A number of things appear to have been happening around the same time that sleep is first revealed on the evolutionary stage, and it may well be that sleep is only one facet of these significant changes. A big change in energy management was underway. Unlike reptiles, a furry and a feathered animal type appeared that could maintain its activity in cold weather, because its brain had acquired a thermostatic mechanism to turn up heat production when the external temperature had dropped. This device opened up a whole new market for these animals . . . the nighttime. Reptiles and maybe dinosaurs (some of which may have been warm-blooded), though not asleep, tended to get stuporous from the evening cold. After about midnight (22:00 hours, dinosaur time, since the earth rotated more rapidly several hundred million years ago), cold-blooded animals were not able to move or react so speedily. This left the wee hours, by default, to the warm-blooded ones. However, maneuvering by night required more reliance on hearing than the highly visual reptiles. Adaptive expansion of hearing was hindered by the bony confines of the middle ear so that enlargement of the brain, with tie lines into the ear, was the only way to go. It is now generally believed that this enlargement of the brain to accommodate more auditory processing paved the way for the development of the brain's capacity to compare inputs from different sensory modalities and to cross-correlate the data. Reptiles see, hear, smell, and feel, but, as some have pointed out, there is apparently no central area for the rapid comparison of these various senses in the brain itself. To be sure, the reptile brain does react to all the sensory input at an "emotional level," but it lacks a cortex to do cognitive processing. As strange as it sounds, it may be argued that a cold-blooded animal is capable of feeling but not thinking. Part of what the mammal does with its cortex (by far the largest part of its brain) is to assemble the various sensory messages from outside into a coherent internal blueprint of what is going on outside. With the capacity to form such internal images came the possibility to store and reproduce them in the form of memory or dreams. If a reptile did sleep, any dreams it might have would most likely be so fragmentary that they would even make Sigmund Freud's head spin.

At this point, one is tempted to speculate that sleep, which seems to make its first appearance during the transition from reptile to mammal, may be a function of brain size. Perhaps the greatly enlarged brain of the mammal needs this special form of rest and recuperation. Since it has much more image processing and memory work to perform (and, as we shall see, the brain remains very active during most phases of sleep), sleeping and dreaming may be the phase of the animal's 24-hour day during which record-keeping and accounting functions are most efficiently performed.

However, sleep is not the exclusive province of brains with an enlarged cortex. Birds, whose brains perform in a manner to justify the perjorative "birdbrain," also sleep. There is considerable evidence that birds are the direct descendants of dinosaurs and, like their forebears, do not have a lot of smarts. The brain of a bird, like that of a reptile, does not appear equipped to do extensive processing of internalized images. Like the reptile, it watches silent movies, listens to records, tastes and feels in separate ways. So to speak, it does not see what it hears nor hear what it sees. If such a low-brained creature sleeps, then what common feature is there to explain the rise of sleep in large-brained mammals and pea-brained birds?

One possible answer is that both are **warm** brains. So, too, are reptile brains at midday and peak activity, but the brains of mammals and birds, unlike those of reptiles, never have a chance to cool off. In fact, many mammals have devised special cooling blood vessel networks to prevent the brain from dangerously overheating. In place of the natural cool-down that would take place in reptiles each night, sleep might be a gear-down phenomenon to take some of the constant heat load off the warm-blooded animal's brain. The brain in man consumes about 20 percent of the blood supply, suggesting an upwards of fiftyfold higher energy consumption and heat generation per ounce than the average for the rest of the body. It would seem that there is little else that bird and mammal brains have in common when compared to reptile brains. The bird, like the reptile, did not develop a large capacity for processing sound, possibly because it could range both day and night in the air, far out of reach of possible enemies. An obvious exception to this is the ostrich, an earthbound bird with a far more intelligent gaze than your average bird, with increased auditory capacity to match.

So sleep may have begun as a local heat control mechanism for the brain and then developed other attributes. Evolution, like General Motors, seems to be a tinkerer rather than a grand redesigner. As each new technological advance is added, remnants of the old hang on in the new design, and often, a new feature turns out to be an old mechanism reworked. As Carl Sagan, among others, has suggested, sleep and its attendant dreaming may have started as a heat control device, only to find further usefulness as a protective inhibition of daytime activity in small mammals during the age of the dinosaur. That this latter use would be a secondary rather than a primary function of sleep is suggested by its presence in the far less vulnerable birds.

Once in place in a somewhat large-brained early mammal, sleep might have then proved a means for still further enlargement of the brain. Using the analogy of a small business where record-keeping is at a minimum, one invariably finds a growth in paperwork, accounting and record-keeping that is out of proportion to the absolute increase in the size of the business. This is not to be dismissed as just a cynical view of the inevitability of "bureaucratization," because as departments develop, the need for regular communication among these subdivisions leads to larger and larger investments in information storage and update. If one department gets too far out in front of the others, as General Patton did with respect to his colleagues in World War II, chaos threatens. More and more time is required to keep all departments up to date. As evolutionary time unfolded and the brain grew larger in successive species under competitive pressure, the break period of sleep might more and more have come to represent an absolutely necessary time for information update. Whether this might be especially true of that division of the sleep cycle during which dreaming primarily occurs, or whether other components of the sleep cycle (during which a hormone, which functions as a stimulant to bodily growth and restoration, is secreted by the brain) play a role in information sorting and consolidation, remains to be established.

There is, however, an intriguing suggestion that people may require more sleep after intensive learning situations. And, of course, babies, who sleep and dream the majority of time, are adding to their information base at the most rapid rate at any time in their lives. Lest we fall victim to some self-serving entrepreneur who creatively reworks this last observation and claims that his audio tapes provide "painless learning while you sleep," we must note that such schemes, loosely based on a simplistic understanding of subliminal phenomena, offer no competitive threat to daytime classes at the Berlitz School.

The above speculation regarding a scenario depicting the evolution of sleep can be summarized as follows: First, the brain develops a body heat control mechanism. As a result, a new, nighttime ecological market opens up. Then, the brain enlarges to allow for improved hearing and smell. A centralized enlargement of sensory processing leads to the cross-correlation of senses with the development of internalized images which more accurately reflect the outside world. In this scenario, sleep is adopted as a primary brain heat control mechanism. Secondarily, sleep becomes a mechanism to keep mammals out of danger during the daytime. Finally, sleep, in the form of REM sleep, permits time for sorting out the day's experiences, now stored in considerable detail within the much larger brain.

It should be kept in mind that it is not unusual for an

evolutionary development to be stood on its head, so to speak, and, like the proverbial resewn and darned sock that contains none of its original wool, to be devoted mainly or exclusively to a function entirely different from the original one. The most dramatic example of this occurred in an earlier epoch when life arose in an essentially oxygen-free atmosphere. During the billions of years of initial evolution, the oxygen level gradually rose to the point where it became possible for multicellular life to develop, leading to the proliferation of all the life forms we know today. Life originally hated oxygen in its free form, and now can rarely do without it (although free oxygen is still a poison to some of those anaerobic forms of bacteria that persist today).

So here we have a series of first-generation speculations regarding the nature and function of sleep. Investigators engage in this kind of informed theorizing not just because such speculation is enjoyable, but also because it is a challenge to further investigation. Consequently, researchers began to look at the regulation of both temperature and sleep.

Although body temperature follows a diurnal rhythm which is independent of the sleep cycle, the timing of sleep has been shown by a research team headed by Charles Czeisler to be linked to the timing of the circadian body temperature rhythm. Specifically, subjects slept longer if they entered sleep at the peak of their temperature cycle as compared with entering sleep at the nadir of that cycle. Since body temperature and alertness are positively correlated, someone entering sleep at the trough of his temperature cycle will only be asleep a short time until his body temperature begins its climb along the ascending limb of its cycle. In other words, these investigators found that the duration of a bout of sleep is correlated not with the amount of presleep wakefulness imposed on the subject, but rather with the rhythmic phase of the body temperature cycle at the time of going to sleep.

HIBERNATION AND THE COORDINATION OF BIORHYTHMS

It is known that associated with stage 4 sleep is a downturned setting of the thermostat that regulates body temperature. This regulator is located in that area of the brain called the hypothalamus. Two additional sleep-related phenomena, estivation (or shallow torpor) and hibernation (or deep torpor), are associated with the down-regulation of body temperature as well. It would seem that both estivation and hibernation make it possible for some warm-blooded animals to adapt to intermittant restrictions in energy provisions available in their environments by lowering their body temperature (and attendant metabolism) to near ambient conditions. Shallow torpor is characterized by a 5°–15°C drop in body temperature, a sleep-like posture, and decreased reactivity to the outside world. It occurs within the regular daily sleep cycle and is present in a number of birds and many small mammals. Hibernation is nowhere near as common. It is characterized by a more marked temperature drop, a more pronounced fall in responsiveness to external stimuli, and a duration that can last over many days with brief awakenings intervening periodically during the cold months of the year. Incidentally, bears are not true hibernators. They, along with some chipmunks and the raccoon for instance, undergo a type of seasonal quiesence called "winter dormancy" or "seasonal sleep" in which body temperature and responsiveness to external stimuli are both maintained at near-normal levels.

Recognition that sleep (in particular, stage 4 or slow wave sleep), like estivation and hibernation, is accompanied by decreases in body temperature and arousal stimulus sensitivity, coupled with studies of the EEG patterns in all three conditions, has led to the understanding that shallow torpor and hibernation are entered via sleep. Furthermore, it was felt that the three phenomena might represent related, perhaps even homologous, processes that lie in sequence along a continuum of increasing dormancy coupled with decreasing body metabolism and temperature, as an organism might move from alertness to slumber, to shallow torpor or hibernation.

With regard to energy factors that might regulate these processes once they have begun, there is evidence to suggest that products of metabolism such as glucose or free fatty acids (critical products derived from the metabolism of lipids and essential for the biochemistry of many different bodily functions) may be involved in regulating the amount and depth of dormancy behaviors. For instance, it has been found that both the total amount of sleep and the distribution of this sleep throughout the 24-hour day can be changed by altering energy metabolites. Normal human subjects on a fast will decrease their total sleep time while slightly increasing their percentage of stage 4 sleep. Both sleep and eating behavior are circadian events which are capable of being shaped by the light–dark cycles of the environment. The manner in which this occurs is as follows: Environmental light strikes the retina of the eye and resultant neuronal impulses are carried down the retinohypothalamic tract (a path of nerve cell fibers so-named for both their origin and destination) to that busy crossroads in the center of the brain, the hypothalamus. There, in a colony of nerve cells called the suprachiasmatic nucleus, the impulses reach what is considered to be the internal oscillator or metronome, in charge of synchronizing many of the body's circadian cyclical functions. From here, neuronal linkages go to another area deep in the brain and less than one-fourth of an inch in diameter, called the epiphysis, or pineal gland (after its pinecone shape). The pineal gland was thought by the 17th century philosopher René Descartes to be the "seat of the soul" or by certain eastern philosophers to represent the "third" or "inner" eye. It is here that the polypeptide hormone melatonin is made and secreted in a rhythm keyed to the cycle of light and darkness. Specifically, the synthesis and secretion of this hormone occurs only during the darkness of night. And this is true for both diurnal and nocturnal animals.

It is believed that melatonin functions as a grand coordinator for a number of endocrine functions elsewhere in the body. Bright sunlight seems to have the potential for habituating, or entraining, physiological functions by suppressing melatonin via the neuronal pathways delineated above. This is suggested by findings demonstrating that exposure to bright light, after jet air travel, can facilitate the re-entrainment of circadian rhythms, or that infertility is more common in blind women, or that in the northernmost reaches of Scandinavia, conceptions occur more commonly during summertime.

To return to our discussion of the interweaving of sleep, eating behavior, and energy conservation as circadian events: As previously mentioned, both eating and sleeping are capable of accommodating to, and in fact are entrainable by, time cues as reflected in the presence or absence of daylight . . . that is, the so-called photoperiod. Sleeping and eating are further associated with circadian shifts between the synthesis and metabolic breakdown of critical body fats or lipids. All this again raises the topic of the putative connection between energy conservation and sleep mechanisms, establishes an understanding of some of the physiological issues, and sets the stage for our subsequent exploration, in Chapter 5, of the interweaving of nutritional factors and sleep events. In this regard, central nervous system neurons that produce the chemical neurotransmitter serotonin (a biochemical relative of melatonin, by the way) play important roles in the regulation of a number of different physiological processes, including the regulation of sleep, body temperature, sexuality, and response to pain and aggression. They also influence the onset and termination of hibernation. It is not clear to what extent this last effect is related to the influence of serotonin directly on a mechanism responsible for control of the hibernating state, or if it is an indirect consequence of the suppressant effect of serotonin on the temperature regulation system. In the latter case, lowering of the body temperature, even beyond the point normally present in deep sleep, would provide the impetus for entry into hibernation.

From studies of sleep, torpor, and hibernation comes the conclusion that the occurrence of these different forms of "dormancy" depends on the presence of factors such as external food supplies, body fat reserves, body size, and environmental conditions such as ambient temperature, and on whether one is predator or prey. Although many people sleep poorly in the cold, not all do. If push comes to shove, we apparently can tap some primordial connection within ourselves and enter unusual states of dormancy. For example, Australian aborigines, living on limited diets, can sleep naked next to small fires at temperatures close to freezing. Under these circumstances, they are able to reduce their body temperatures and, in effect, enter the state of shallow torpor which had been thought to be reserved only for small mammals and birds. Upon arousal, they are reported to warm themselves in a way similar to that used by animals arising from a long winter hibernation . . . shivering violently, and then going about their business.

Sleep and its related phenomena are highly complicated processes. What is the function of sleep? What roles do its subdivisions serve? Why is the process so intricate? Answers to these questions are not yet available with any degree of certainty. For that matter, it is not even known what the objective or operative target of sleep is and whether the brain, in the words of the endocrinologist, is its end-organ. Since sleep does take time, and it takes time away from other vital undertakings (like feeding and vigilance), it is assumed to be instrumental in important biological business. But if the purpose of sleep is to replenish and to restore, we do not know yet what is being replenished or what is being restored.

Chapter 3

From Stuffed Teddies to Hot Toddies

Sleep in the Young and Sleep in the Old

"I had a good night's sleep!" We have often heard that phrase but what, in fact, does it mean? That you are well rested? Well, no, because you can lie in bed, awake but resting, and a whole night of this calm repose will still leave you sleepy in the morning. So it is more than just bodily or physical rest that must be involved.

If you were to witness the phenomenon of sleep from the outside, like an alien observer from Mars, you might assume that sleep is but a passive response to the environmental cyclical factors of light and darkness. But we have already established that sleep is not a simple and uniform state of physiological inactivity, providing only time out until the next rising of the sun. Rather, sleep is composed of a number of highly organized and coordinated activities involving the nervous, muscular, vascular, and endocrine gland systems. With periodic operations like 90-minute REM cycles, cycles of secretion of chemicals (like prolactin and growth hormone from the endocrine glands) reaching crescendos during each NREM phase, periodic flare-ups of skin electrical activity, and four or five penile erections occurring throughout the night (even in young children, and continuing into old age, as long as no medical complication intervenes), it is in fact mind-boggling to realize just how complex, let alone how busy, the phenomenon of sleep really is.

Although there is no consensus about what makes up a normal night's sleep, there are generally agreed upon parameters, the outer limits of which are considered abnormal. Sleep patterns offer a wide range of the "normal," between different individuals, as well as within each individual at different times in his or her life history, so that clearcut choices between what is to be considered normal and what is not are not always easily decided. Additionally, not only do individual characteristics vary, but so too do individuals' expectations of what will be considered "normal." Specifically, an individual's subjective judgment of the nature of his or her sleep is very susceptible to outside influences, be they changes in internal state or inputs from external sources. As a result, by the way, one's subjective judgment about the quality of sleep is a notoriously inaccurate reflection of true sleep duration and/or disturbance, when compared with objective measurements of sleep done in the sleep lab.

As we have established, the state of sleep is neither inactive nor homogeneous. It is characterized by the presence of a distinctive and varied pattern of events, recurring on a cyclical basis, and called the sleep architecture. Through electronic monitoring of brain waves (using the EEG), eye movements (using the electrooculogram or EOG), and muscle tone (using the electromyogram or EMG), one can watch the behavioral progression from wakefulness to sleep and track the physiological transitions, first between the lighter stages (1 and 2) of sleep to the deeper ones, and then on to REM sleep. One can follow the changes in voltage, amplitude and configuration of the tracings on the EEG characteristic for each stage of sleep. Furthermore, we can follow, in parallel, the activity of the respiratory and circulatory systems through the sleep cycle. If we do, we will note the consistent decline in respiratory rate, pulse rate and blood pressure during NREM sleep, while these same measures show marked and apparently erratic fluctuations during the REM state.

CHARACTERISTICS OF NORMAL SLEEP

So what characterizes normal sleep? For one, it is less the absolute total duration of sleep (which, as mentioned, varies from individual to individual and with different ages over the lifespan of each individual) and more the consistency from night to night with regard to the proportion of time spent in each sleep stage. Sleep patterns, like fingerprints, remain reasonably characteristic for each individual, and maintain a stability throughout the young adult and middle-age adult years, as long as no extraordinarily intrusive circumstances intervene. There are, however, certain qualities of sleep patterns which are peculiar to specific epochs of life. So let us look at an overview of the evolution of sleep over a lifetime, and trace the changes which occur in the general features of sleep as we age.

The average total length of sleep of the newborn is 16 hours. It is spread out in multiple episodes over the 24-hour day. By puberty, the total sleep time is down to about 8 hours a night, from which it eventually levels off to about 7 hours a night during the adult middle years. Then, a gradual decline in average total sleep time of about 30 minutes or so creeps in during the "senior" years, along with an increased fragmentation of sleep (with more frequent awakenings and more difficulty returning to sleep). The duration of sleep latency (that is, the time needed to fall asleep) gradually increases with increasing age.

As an individual ages into the senior years, easy arousal from sleep by noise or other environmental perturbations becomes more pronounced and as a result, there is an increase in daytime sleepiness and napping. Time spent in bed increases although the ability to get to sleep, and therefore the efficiency of the sleeping process, gradually decreases. Additionally, the amount of stages 3 and 4, comprising "delta" or "deep" sleep, decreases and a less prominent but still significant reduction in REM sleep occurs. Finally, the elderly comes to gradually experience a shift in the sleep–wake cycle to earlier hours, leading to what has been called the "advanced phase syndrome." Here, the bedtime hours occur ever earlier, the person still has difficulty getting up in the morning, and the actual circadian sleep–wake rhythm slips into an ultradian one of 22 to 23 hours in duration. Coupled with this phase shift is an increased intolerance to other imposed phase shifts. An example is jet lag: long distance travel becomes more and more difficult for us to adjust to as we get older. Incidentally, the opposite syndrome to "advanced phase" is called "phase delayed." It can be seen during weekdays in younger individuals who have slightly reset their body clocks during the weekends by staying up late. They experience the consequences of this during the week when they encounter difficulty going to sleep at night and then waking up the following morning.

JET LAG

As long as we are talking about phase shifts and the timing of cycles, let us look more closely at the phenomenon of jet lag. It is an occurrence that is very much a part of the natural order of things, given our ability to transgress time zones now in a way that was probably not anticipated, during the early stages of Creation, while we were still on the drawing board. To begin our discussion, we must first return to the relationship among sleep cycles, body temperature and energy metabolism.

A number of investigators, Moore-Ede, Weitzman, Kronauer, and Czeisler, who were co-workers at Montefiore Hospital in New York City, substantiated the claim of the intimate interplay between body temperature and other body rhythms (Moore-Ede, 1986). Core body temperature goes through a regular daily ebb and flow, starting from an early morning low point and gradually rising to a high in the mid-afternoon at 2:00 PM, only to gradually recede to the early morning low again, at about 2:00 AM. The specific point in this temperature cycle during which a person goes to sleep will determine the duration of sleep. Previously, common wisdom had it that the amount of time awake prior to going to sleep determines the length of the sleep session. Not so.

We usually go to bed as our body temperature cycle is sloping downward toward its 2:00 AM nadir and, as such, we sleep for approximately 7 hours. When the Montefiore researchers tested individuals, in a sleep lab, who went to sleep at the height of their body temperature cycle (at about 2:00 PM, under usual conditions), they found that these subjects slept for twice as many hours! And they were able to replicate this effect outside the lab, in the real world, just as long as the attempt to sleep was preceded by a significant amount of time (about 14 hours) spent awake so that there was at least an urge to sleep. Put another way, if you stay up burning the midnight oil and then try to catch a few winks early in the morning, say at 6:00 AM, you will sleep relatively briefly, rising, in effect, with your rising temperature cycle (and it is tempting to speculate that this phenomenon underlies that reliable but elusive internal alarm clock that so many are blessed with or, alternatively, can't seem to shake). But if you can hold out until early afternoon before trying to "catch up," you may well find yourself sleeping right through the night to your normal waking time the next morning. The effects of cycles are indeed profound.

So what happens when we tinker with them by flying to distant shores? We face the by now familiar phenomenon of jet lag. By rapidly changing time zones (with the attendant changes in social and environmental cues by which our own cycles have been entrained), we place demands on our timing systems to acclimate to the new surroundings. Our pacemakers have the elasticity to do this but their pace is slow. We can indeed gradually adjust to such time shifts by about one hour per day. But there are inherent limits to the resetting of the circadian system clocks so that we cannot maintain a forced disruption far from the 24-hour periodicity for very long without incurring seriously disordering consequences. With regard to jet flight, the gradual adjustment to the new time cues is more rapid when the circadian rhythms must slow down relative to the time in the new environment—that is, when flying from east to west. In an analogous way, those late sleepers on weekends are trifling with rhythms somewhat like the world traveler. They go to bed later and sleep later, creating an effect akin to that which would be gotten flying from west to east. They then come back to earth on Monday, with a morning-after befuddlement. Are such phase shifts the basis for the Monday "blues"? Does a specific shifting of circadian cycles on the weekend account not just for these "blahs" but also for the anticipatory anxiety experienced by some on Sunday, the evening before? And what about all those who, either for work-related reasons (like submarine crewmen, transcontinental pilots, or shift workers such as hospital interns), or environmental circumstances (like dwellers in the northern reaches of the Arctic Circle), or because of physiological influences (associated with the likes of pregnancy or adolescence), are in a more or less persistent state of "circadian instability"? Are there not ways in which we might be able to more specifically anticipate and address the behavioral and physiological consequences of such conditions? The answers to these questions remain to be determined, but the foundation for understanding, upon which these answers will rest, has begun to be established.

SLEEP AND BODY TEMPERATURE

In any case, body temperature and energy metabolism seem to be intimately related to the processes that set the timing of sleep. If this is true, and as the metabolic fires burn ever longer, then perhaps there occurs a fall off in the total amount of sleep (usually at the expense of stage 4 NREM sleep and REM sleep) and a fragmentation of what sleep there is, as the body-building, heat-conserving, sleep-promoting years of youth give way to the catabolic fires of old age. Whether this can be used as a literal model of aging (that is, of catabolic breakdown and heat loss) is doubtful, but it does suggest a theoretical structure within which to catalogue the following observations regarding sleep, energy metabolism, and aging. Hypothermia, which results from the profound chilling that can occur in those stranded in ice and snow, leads to an urge to sleep. Additionally, as noted above, we tend to sleep during the times of our lowest body temperatures (during which our sense of alertness also seems to be at its lowest) and tend to rise as this temperature begins to rise. With regard to REM sleep, it is interesting to note the coordination of the body's lowest temperature point with the timing of the most prominent REM episode of the night. And finally, with aging, there seems to be a change in the coordination and timing of temperature cycles and sleep which appears to be related to gender differences.

Regarding this last point, according to Campbell and his colleagues (1989), elderly women show more changes in temperature cycles than elderly men, with lower baseline temperatures and more volatile changes from highs to lows throughout the course of the evening. Whatever the mechanisms underlying such a finding might be (be they related to a hormonal, psychological or another, as yet unidentified mechanism), it is probably too simplistic to suggest that they account for the observation made by some that: (1) with couples, at least in our society, it is the woman who appears to be more sensitive to the cold, and (2) women are twice as likely to complain of insomnia as men. Reynolds and his colleagues (1986) have documented the fact that elderly men and women respond differently to a bout of sleep deprivation, with women exhibiting, on average, a more pronounced increase in recovery sleep following the deprivation than do men. Furthermore women, again on average, appear to show more mood disturbances after such deprivation than their male counterparts do. Is there, embedded in these impressionistic claims (and supported to some extent by surveys, formal and informal) and controlled studies, a basis for connecting the effects of body temperature and sleep cycles to each other? In order to begin to answer this question, one of the things that needs to be tested is the extent to which the manipulation of external temperature can in a predictable and reliable way affect the nature and characteristics of sleep in both men and women.

One final speculative point regarding the interactions among body temperature, energy utilization, and sleep, before returning to our characterization of the "normal" sleep cycle which we left before. The psychological occasion of "anxiety" is associated with the physiological event of increased adrenaline secretion. The catecholamine, adrenaline, is an interesting substance that aids in arousing the body at times of threatened danger. It also encourages the metabolic breakdown of bodily material to release energy, presumably needed during heightened states of alert and alarm. Additionally, perhaps as part of this "catabolic" activity, it causes body temperature to rise. Hence we possibly have a mechanism by which anxiety can interfere with sleep, operating through channels that closely link temperature and sleep cycles. Furthermore, we have a basis from which to hypothesize about the sleep-inducing properties of aspirin that are claimed by some. The pharmacist will insist it is not a hypnotic agent; however, aspirin lowers body temperature and, under certain circumstances, as we have just seen, decreased temperature is associated with increased sleepiness. The seesawing interplay among the variety of factors involved with body rhythmic cycles can indeed be indirect, curious, and at times, surprising. Their actions in concert result in the profile we have of normal sleep patterns.

SLEEP AND NIGHTTIME INTERRUPTIONS

But how do we determine what a normal sleep episode is? Afterall, how many sleep environments can guarantee no intrusions? And if there is an interruption, do occasional or brief intrusions have lasting effects on sleep characteristics? From the crashing of garbage pails in the alley, to the crying of a newborn in the middle of the night, it is certainly clear that the structure of sleep can be modified by increasing environmental perturbations. The question asked more systematically is: What happens to sleep after a forced, unanticipated, or unusual awakening? What happens to the subsequent duration of sleep and to the architecture of the sleep cycle?

Of course many issues come into play here, and many factors have to be taken into account. But an interesting study by a group of French investigators headed by Foret (1990) determined that when a significant interruption occurred during the night, it had no noticeable effect on subsequent sleep structure. Whether interruptions took place early in the sleep cycle or sometime later on seemed to make no difference in the subsequent duration of the sleep episode. And yet these researchers were aware of apparently contradictory findings which reported that sleep cycles are indeed prolonged following interruptions in the cycle, and that sleep architecture can change as a result of such interruptions. How were they to reconcile these claims with their observations?

For an answer, Foret's team looked within the sleep cycle, at the specific timing of the interruption. They found that if the interruption occurred during NREM sleep, very little subsequent effect was noted. But imposed awakenings occurring during the REM cycle had profound effects. They discovered that, following REM sleep interruption, the total duration of the next REM cycle was significantly reduced in length. They speculated that this may reflect a resetting of the neurological mechanisms that time the REM cycle and switch it on. Their model can be likened to an electric gate mechanism which opens automatically, by engaging an electric motor and a mechanical clutch, once the magnetic card "key" has been inserted into the opening slot. The sequence proceeds in an orderly fashion, from initial signal through the starting of the motor, to the engagement of the clutch, and the opening of the gate; then a pause in the open position, and the subsequent swinging close with a culminating, quiet disengagement. But what if the card, having just initiated the sequence, is suddenly reintroduced in midstream, sending in another signal superimposed on the cycle already in progress? Well, depending on when in the cycle that additional, interrupting signal is introduced, it will either be ignored, stall the entire process, or be incorporated into the sequence in such a way as to lead to the starting point again (either through a rapid phase-advance to the beginning, or a retreat and return to "square one"). In a somewhat analogous way, we may view the effects that brief sleep interruptions may have, when introduced during REM sleep, on the overall profile of sleep patterns. As a corollary, some have suggested that the very timing of REM sleep sets the pattern of the total sleep cycle, with NREM sleep just filling in the gaps.

PATTERNS OF SLEEP OVER A LIFETIME

When wrestling with definitions of what is "normal," we inevitably come across categories of traits that form continua rather than discrete clear-cut categories. Early on in sleep research, characteristics such as habitual bedtime, pliancy and resilience of sleep habits, and differences in the timing of peaks of performance efficiency, were anchored by two extremes of what was considered to be the spectrum of normalcy—night "owls" and day "larks." It most certainly is true that many basic behavioral traits, like sex-specific behaviors, sleep patterns, and cognitive styles, are founded on core neurobiological qualities comprising phenomena such as gender-related traits and temperament. Is the same true for the sleep cycle traits of the larks and owls? Certainly, people living in similar environments, with similar demands and social behaviors, show individual differences in their sleep–wake cycles, just like they show differences in their hair color or body weight.

But inputs from core qualities, such as those just mentioned, are filtered through a sieve of parental interaction and responsiveness early on and, later, through the screen of broader social interaction and pressure. The "fit" between the maturing individual and his/her parents, and then between the individual and other aspects of the environment, is of critical importance in determining the direction that developing behaviors will take. To what extent social pressure and the development of certain habits has led to the evolution of specific temperaments—like the "morning person" or his "evening" counterpart, as opposed to the preordained temperament type dictating the kind of sleep habits and profiles that will prevail—remains to be seen. Initial exploration into this area, however, has determined that the morning lark and the evening owl are indistinguishable from each other with regard to body temperature cycles or REM sleep characteristics.

From a behavioral point of view, it is not clear whether the reinforcement that supports a particular behavior, such as the sleep cycle in humans, is related to:

1. a specific developmental event (like parental responsiveness)
2. a specific substance (like a neurotransmitter or a hormone)
3. the very operation of a neurophysiological process with its attendant behavioral sequences
4. other factors, working separately or in combination

With respect to the third factor, let us reconfirm our understanding that there are many kinds of fixed, repetitive action patterns, which we are calling "cycles," that are set by the biological structure of our very essences. Such "wired in" patterns, encompassing the likes of mating, sleeping, and, perhaps, fighting behaviors, have terminating stimuli which are reinforcing. In mating, it can be orgasm. In fighting, in particular with mammals other than man, it can be the so-called "surrender response," which occurs when one animal clearly dominates the other: the loser withdraws and the winner does not pursue, so that further physical struggle is averted. And in sleeping . . . well here we are

less sure. We do know that, as we mature and accumulate experience, a whole set of behaviors becomes established, related to
biologically driven cycles such as eating or sleeping. We hypothesize that when such cyclical patterns of behavior are brought to
completion, there results a state which is inherently positive and
reinforcing. From this, then, develop recurrent expectancies, associated thoughts and connections to various social and time cues.

But the answer to the question of what the specific reinforcing
factors are is complicated. These factors are varied, involved, and
interwoven. As just one example of this complexity, breast-fed
babies tend to maintain their track of nighttime wakings longer
than bottle-fed babies. But they too tend to stop this pattern with
weaning, suggesting that the nighttime contact, more than the
feeding schedule or some specific quality of the milk alone, is
important. Additionally, perhaps because of temperamental differences, some sleepless infants cry out while others, the more
sanguine ones, suffer in relative silence.

The pattern of the human sleep cycle is first detected in the
32-week old fetus. At that time, signs of REM sleep first appear,
followed a month or two later by the appearance of NREM sleep. A
premature infant spends about 80 percent of its sleep time in
REM sleep while a full-term newborn spends 50 percent. During
the first months of infancy, the REM stage initiates sleep, and
periods of REM sleep occur more frequently than in the adult
(about every 60 minutes rather than every 90 minutes). The
overall structure of sleep evolves from an amorphous mix of sleep
and wake time in the newborn, to a more formed pattern, at about
9 months of age, when the relatively equal distribution of "active"
sleep (the precursor of REM sleep) and "quiet" sleep (the germinal
state of NREM sleep) changes throughout the night. Now the
apportionment of sleep stages first begins to take on more of the
pattern that we will eventually see in the adult: REM sleep loaded
more toward the end of the sleep cycle and NREM sleep (in
particular, stages 3 and 4) more toward the beginning. But it is not
until approximately 4 years of age that a true, diurnal, biphasic
rhythm of sleeping and waking is established. And it is at this age
that REM sleep comes to make up the 20 percent component of
sleep time that will be its continued allotment into adulthood.

As the infant's sleep pattern begins to regularize and congeal into a form more reflective of the adult picture, the duration of night sleep at first increases, from 6–8 hours at age 4 months, to 10–12 hours by 6 months of age. Most infants sleep a total of 16–20 hours a day for the first 6 months of life, and by 6 months most can sleep through the night. By 2 years of age, the average child sleeps 12–14 hours a day. This total sleep time gradually decreases thereafter but, throughout the pediatric age range, does not fall below 10 hours of sleep a night.

It is common for up to one-third of all children aged 1–3 years to be reluctant to go to sleep. Most observers of child psychological development feel that this is related to a normal growth stage in which the child begins to establish a sense of mastery of his/her own by undertaking to separate from the parents. It is the time of the protests and the "no's," the "terrible two's." But as necessary for development as these pulls and urges toward autonomy are, they are equally frightening. This developmental "dilemma," a part of everyone's growing up, is thought to lead to what has been called "separation anxiety," a phenomenon which reflects both the attraction of developing an individual personality distinct from the influential inputs of one's overseers, and, on the other side of the coin, the fear of abandonment and annihilation that might come from this same loss of the protective parental umbrella. As the child's ability to conceptualize improves, he will be better able to hold on to images of the parents from whom he temporarily separates so that he can maintain a sense of continuity that will sustain him during these actual periods of separation from people and objects to whom he has been attached.

In this context, it can be appreciated that sleep itself may be viewed as a "separation" from the concrete personages of the waking world and, to the vulnerable youngster contending with these developmental demands, as a state to be avoided. Helpful, transitional sleep time "crutches" are normal during this period, and include the Teddy Bear, or a favorite blanket, or that perennial favorite, from which he is literally inseparable, the thumb.

Many preschoolers take a long time going to sleep and demand that a light be left on. In addition to the normal developmental consideration just mentioned, children can experience some delay in going to sleep for a number of reasons. These include the presence of physical illness, primary sleep disorders, or environmental disruptions, as well as psychological issues revolving around nighttime feedings or haphazard limit-setting by the parents.

In any case, it must be reemphasized that there is a certain amount of latitude to the concept of "normal," and what is abnormal for one individual or group of children may be within the normal range for another. For instance, nighttime bedwetting and daytime naps are normal in the youngest children but not so by age of seven or eight. By the same token, an occasional episode of night terror or sleepwalking (which will be discussed more fully in Chapter 9) may be normal in the young child, if it is indeed infrequent and not overly intense. Certain bedtime rhythmic movements like body rocking or stereotyped head rolling or banging (called *jactatio capitio nocturna* and, oddly enough, a variant of sleep-related behavior) can likewise be normal concomitants of sleep in children, just as long as they are not too violent nor last longer than 15 minutes or so. Of course, these movements can also be seen in emotionally disturbed or developmentally retarded children, but other signs and symptoms clue us in to the presence of these conditions.

Other sleep behaviors reported by parents, that are common and therefore presumed to be within the bounds of normalcy, include restlessness, complaints about not being able to sleep, and smiling and laughing during sleep. Fisher and colleagues (1989) surveyed parents to establish normative data on the sleep behavior of children up to the sixth grade. As part of this survey, they determined that, within certain limits, sleep traits were not affected by the number of siblings nor by the rank in birth order of the particular child.

When we turn our attention to teenagers, we see a rather consistent picture emerge . . . that of increased daytime sleepiness and decreased nighttime sleep. But what lies behind such a change? A decreased need to sleep? A lessening in the ability to sleep? Or increased social pressure to stay awake? Strauch and Meier (1988) suggest from their study that adolescents frequently long for more sleep but find that they express this desire inconsistently, depending on who is listening and what the social options are that are pressing. As we will discuss later on, the current interest in finding us all "sleep-deprived" has gained much popular coverage in the press. But getting less sleep is not necessarily the same as being "sleep-deprived." For one thing, some people just need less sleep. Additionally, the significance of a small, although not unimportant subgroup of chronically "poor" sleepers, who seem to need less sleep, is not known. And further, one can see little in the way of functional impairment in healthy volunteers subjected to experimental sleep loss. In fact, it is not until about 60 hours of sleep loss has occurred that significant distortions in mental functioning start to be seen. Only at that rather extreme point can illusions and hallucinations begin to appear, superimposed on the sleepiness and decreased ability to concentrate that had already been established. And even with 60 hours of sleep deprivation, there seems to be little deleterious effect on one's aerobic capacity and efficiency during exercise. Whether this is due to the fact that sleep loss has no affect on oxygen utilization during exertion, or rather that the arousal concomitant with aerobic exercise overwhelms the dampening effects of loss, has yet to be determined.

While we are discussing "sleep deprivation," let's make one point about sleep duration, either too long or too short. A survey of 1 million adults, conducted through the University of California at San Diego in 1979, implied a link between "death expectancy" and sleep duration. Earlier surveys by other organizations suggested an increased mortality rate among men and women who slept less than 4 hours or more than 10 hours. We will discuss more of this in Chapter 4 but let us just note, for the record, that the significance of such statistics is not understood as yet and certainly does not imply that, merely by extending the sleep of brief sleepers or by arousing long sleepers earlier, you can prolong life. It would be interesting to determine whether there is a difference between these two groups in terms of memory functions, creativity, or dream recall because, as we will discuss in Chapter 5, REM sleep has been implicated by some investigators in many of these functions, and, by definition, long sleepers may spend relatively more time in REM sleep than short sleepers. Conversely, since the total sleep episode of the short sleepers is truncated, perhaps this group suffers a specific and proportionately larger loss of REM sleep.

In any case, "early to bed, early to rise" appears to be the hallmark of the young child and the elderly, certainly not the adolescent and the young adult. During middle adolescence, into the college years, time spent sleeping decreases, only to increase in the middle adult years to maintain the expected 7–8 hours a night range. What accounts for this dip? Certainly adolescents, contending with maturational milestones of both a hormonal and a psychological nature, are known for practices that stretch parental tolerance for irregularity, sleep habits being one of these. And college students, away from home, living in a highly charged communal environment with work and social demands and peer distractions can fall prey to the clarion call of "one more party!" The problem is that, although instigated by social factors, ensuing sleep pattern distortions can take on a life of their own and present the clinician with an adolescent suffering from the "delayed sleep-phase syndrome."

This syndrome comes about in teenagers, for instance, who cannot bring themselves to go to sleep until the wee hours, then sleep normally but cannot delay their rising time. They have to awaken to take care of their day's business. They exhibit extraordinary difficulty in getting up in the morning, and they may have excessive daytime sleepiness, lagging school performance along with school avoidance in some cases (distinguishable from so-called school phobia where the youngster is less interested in recognizing and correcting the underlying problem, and more interested in total avoidance of the school setting), and parents who are beside themselves with frustration.

Thorpy and his co-workers (1988) devised a clever strategy for treating such youngsters in order to get their lives back on track. It is called sleep deprivation with a phase advance (SDPA). It involves an initial baseline sleep schedule maintained for 6 days, followed by one night of no sleep. On the night subsequent to the total sleep deprivation, bedtime and wake time are purposely shifted 90 minutes earlier. The new schedule is maintained for another 6 days, at which time the sleep period is again shifted forward by an additional 90 minutes. By this method, the adolescent's sleep phase is advanced without requiring nights on end spent in the sleep laboratory.

CAUSES OF SLEEP PATTERN CHANGES

In general, we may view falling asleep as being governed by two reciprocally interacting mechanisms. First, there is the "arousal system," which must be turned down low enough to allow sleep to occur. Then there is the "sleep system," which must be activated. Additionally, however, there are mechanisms and systems involved, not in sleep initiation but in sleep maintenance. For, just as there are differences between the ignition system of an automobile and the system that keeps the engine firing once under way, so too the neurobiological machinery of the body is outfitted with many operations, linked in series and in parallel, which oversee its functioning. Given the complexity and diversity of the factors involved, each component of the overall system adds a dimension of latitude, creating a certain leeway in the definition of what would be "normal" for the operation of the system as a whole. Spark plugs fire within a certain specified **range** of timing accuracy; different cylinders, with slightly varying tolerances, operate within a **range** of efficiency; distinct batches of gasoline with slightly dissimilar octane ratings and different amounts of trace contaminants provide a potential energy output, within a **range**, upon combustion. We, similarly, sleep within a **range** of normal.

So what factors account for the variances of sleep patterns? I choose "variance," rather than "normal," to close our discussion here, because so much of what we expect determines our criteria of normalcy that we may be better served by exploring the range of factors that influence our sleep and lead to the varied picture of the phenomenon. Later, in Chapter 9, we will discuss the primary sleep-related disorders.

Although sleeping well after exercise is part of our common lore, research suggests that exercise does not necessarily increase either the total duration of sleep or the amount of NREM "deep" sleep. Furthermore, it is clear that vigorous aerobic exercise can disrupt sleep, as can any intense exercise performed too close to bedtime. Malnutrition and concurrent medical illnesses can both directly and indirectly (through associated symptoms like pain, shortness of breath and urinary frequency) affect sleep patterns, as can the side effects or withdrawal effects of medications taken.

And what about sex? Let us not overlook some of our

commonly-held ideas of the relationship between sexual activity (both with a partner and without one) and sleep. Well, in one of the few attempts made to systematically look at this arena, several investigators in Montreal (Brissette *et al.*, 1985) were able to find no objective effects of either intercourse or masturbation, with or without orgasm, on the structure of sleep. However, if one turns to the subjective and psychological level of inquiry, the results are much more evident, although not necessarily consistent. Some report sleepiness after orgasm while others report increased alertness. The reports further vary depending on concomitant life events and on whether orgasm was achieved in the context of sexual intercourse with a partner or via solitary masturbation. From our mention of sex, we might extend our discussion of factors affecting the dimensions of sleep to include other social and interactional considerations like the behavior, health and habits of one's sleeping partner, be it human, canine, or feline. Hobson and his associates in 1978 were able to document the common-sense notion (simply by taking time-lapse pictures of normal sleepers at home) that there is a close relationship between the sleep behaviors of sleeping partners and that the degree of a sleeper's movement during sleep was correlated with his/her subsequent rating of the "goodness' of that sleep.

Other factors affecting sleep that fall under the category of "interpersonal" include the degree of social and sensory isolation and the psychological reactions triggered by it that have specific effects on sleep organization. Such is the case with depression which, in many of its forms, can distort the sleeping process. An additional example, worthy of mention, is the mother of a newborn infant. Here there are two kinds of tiredness often noted: one, a physical fatigue, which can be relieved by several hours of catch-up sleep; the other, an emotional fatigue related to the responsibility of caring for an infant around the clock, from which there is no respite. This latter phenomenon fits better into the category of "stress" and as such, is relieved by appropriate emotional and physical support.

Finally, let us again note the universal effect of aging on sleep, with its nocturnal phase advance and dissolution of some of the boundaries of sleep architecture. As one ages, the average time taken to fall asleep (sleep latency) more than doubles, the total sleep time (duration) decreases by about 30 minutes, and the average number of awakenings per night (fragmentation) increases from about three to seven or more. The elderly spend the majority of their sleep time in stages 1 and 2 of NREM sleep, relatively little time in stage 4 sleep, and perhaps a slightly reduced amount of time in REM sleep.

Meanwhile, the length of the REM–NREM sleep cycle tends to shorten. With more shifts in sleep stages and more daytime sleepiness, a compensatory attempt is often made to make up for "lost" sleep by spending more time in bed or by napping. And, paradoxically, some may try to counterbalance their daytime sleepiness by increasing their consumption of coffee or tea. With all this comes the recognition that the quality of sleep has changed. In many healthy elderly individuals, this last factor is a key reason for sleep complaints. As with so much that is related to the phenomenon of sleep, the attitudes and expectations, the psychological sets with which one enters the experience, significantly color the outcome. It is therefore important for us, in our exploration of the secrets of sleep, to understand more fully how the neurophysiological brain and psychological behavior are interconnected. In the next chapter we will look at issues regarding the continuity between mind and body as they pertain to the phenomenon of sleep.

Chapter 4

The Elephant and the Blind Men

Various Approaches to the Brain and Behavior . . . Sleep Efficiency and Naps

We human beings are, according to some, examples of an accident of nature: organisms imbued through the eons of evolutionary time with the "chance" of self-awareness and its accoutrements. As a result, and accompanying this unrequested ability to comprehend, we experience that most wonderful of human assets, the drive to master our circumstances. If one seriously considers the bases for these intricate phenomena on anything other than a mystical level of discourse, one must be in awe of the complexity involved, the wonderful intricacy by which these extraordinary events are brought about.

And depending on our starting point and frame of reference, we will each describe the same intricacy somewhat differently, like the blind men, each describing the elephant from his own particular and circumscribed tactile vantage point. Our probing and increasingly deeper exploration of the mysteries of human behavior do not merely entail peeling layer after layer off the problem, like the concentric layers of an onion, until we reach some inner core of truth. Rather, it is more like peeling multiple onions while

simultaneously attempting to see how these different layers relate
to each other.

As our knowledge of the interface between neurological and
psychological function grows, it becomes ever clearer that the
overarching mechanisms which coordinate not only these phenomena, but our daily negotiations through life's gamut of internal and external physical requirements and constraints as well, sit
squarely within the brain. This is true even though we may not yet
be able to point to the specific sites within the agency where each
specific function resides. This organ, this seat of self-awareness
and the drive to ask and to indicate, can construct matrices (ideas)
incorporating previously stored data (memories) along with currently perceived inputs. This brain can rework entries and issue
forth a new product and then reflect upon it, raising new questions. To bend Descartes just a bit: I think, therefore I am . . . I
think!

This is exhausting work. It demands energetic endeavor
against the disordering force of entropy. The heart, like the brain,
but perhaps in a more mundane laborer-like way, also is constantly
at work. How does it pace itself to sustain a lifetime of activity?
Well, like the brain, like the kidneys, like all vital organs, it
functions as if by some inner mandate dictated by its very biological makeup. But it paces itself and utilizes its resources as judiciously as possible while maintaining its duly commissioned responsibilities, regulated by a time-honored biological wisdom
developed over ages of trial and error. Hearts beat, with alternating contractions and relaxation, and brains sleep. But although
asleep, brains still function. From a physiological point of view, this
has become increasingly obvious, as we will discuss more in the
chapter on REM sleep. Other, more psychological, questions arise.
Among these are the following: Given the specific qualities, traits,
and limitations of each individual brain, what factors account for
changes in output and efficiency of brain function? What is the
role of sleep with regard to dimensions of memory, performance,
and creativity? Why can a brief nap be refreshing? Since the
sleeping brain still functions, is it possible to "learn" while we
sleep, once we overcome the sensory barriers raised during the
sleeping state? Does surmounting such thresholds (thereby allowing the registration of inputs normally excluded during the sleeping state) change the very nature of that state? What are the

effects on performance and mentation of changes in sleep characteristics and timing? What is the nature of the interplay between sleep and memory? Or creativity and sleep? Is sleep an incubator of creativity? Is the image of the dreamer as a creator of new illuminations just apocryphal?

As the era of computers permeates our lives more and more, it is not surprising that neuroscientists have turned their attention to this technology to assist in the attempt to develop models of brain and mind activity. Increasingly sophisticated physiological monitoring of brain activity has led to exciting theories regarding the steps underlying human information processing.

Efficient learning obviously requires a functioning brain, intact on many levels. Work with learning-impaired children, especially those with an impaired attention span, has led to an increased appreciation of the role of chemistry in the learning process. Work published at the beginning of the last decade shows that other cognitive skills such as reading, pattern recognition, rhythm, color sense, and analytic and logical capacity can be influenced by fluctuations in the chemical output of certain brain cell populations. More recent work suggests that there may be demonstrable 90-minute swings between right and left brain dominance in ordinary people. What the significance of these swings is for cognitive efficiency and style, and how they interact with sleep–wake states, is by no means clear yet, but we will speak more of this in just a bit.

Finally, it is well known that cognitive performance is impaired in different ways in different psychopathological states. Memory is the chief victim in depression, logic in schizophrenia, and attention in hyperkinetic states—but the degree to which cognitive shifts take place outside of clinically studied conditions is a relatively unscrutinized phenomenon. As always, the study of the sick increases the understanding of the well. The reverse is also true. Sleep researchers, by not drawing an absolute line between sick and healthy, are trying to delineate and illustrate biological mechanisms that are universal. For instance, dreaming—a special cognitive state with certain phenomenological links to psychotic hallucination: The same chemicals that aggravate hallucinations have been shown to enhance the vividness of dreams in nonpsychotic people.

Investigation currently proceeds at different levels of inquiry (from the chemical to the physiological to the psychological), exploring the many dimensions of human information processing. One of the physiological levels of brain function, recently made popular in the lay press, is that referred to by the phrase "cerebral laterality" . . . the so-called left and right brains. Like the two segments of a large walnut, the left and right halves of the cerebral cortex, with its familiar coral-like convoluted surface, sit atop a supporting foundation of densely packed subcortical nerve centers. These subcortical nerve centers, themselves, rest on a column of primal nerve centers called the brainstem, which coordinate and control vital biological functions such as circulation, respiration . . . and sleep. To complete this briefest of tours of the central nervous system, the brainstem then is in continuous connection with the spinal cord, the conduit which provides two-way traffic between the central nervous system and the body's peripheral sense, muscular, and hormonal organs. The fact of the presence of a left and a right half of the cortex (although these are intimately interconnected through a band of linking fibers called the corpus callosum) has raised the question regarding cerebral specialization: Are the different cerebral hemispheres means for the accomplishment of different functions? The brain is a multipurpose organ where many different activities occur. Are there specific anatomical sites for the various agencies regulating the different functional activities, or are the regulatory functions supervising the different activities more diffusely distributed throughout the organ, perhaps just timed to operate on different schedules?

The study of sleep and its disorders is an emerging medical science that cuts across the areas of many other disciplines . . . from the biochemical to the sociological, from the submicroscopic arena of interneuronal chemical messengers to the full-sized world of work shifts and jet lag and their effects on sleep and performance. But changes in sleep, unlike other areas subjected to medicine's search for the pathological, seem functional rather than structural in nature (although the specific nature of the function or functions served by sleep is not yet clear). That is, with rare exception, disorders of human sleep do not seem to represent a mechanical or biochemical disorder localized in one specific area of one particular "organ."

It is necessary to look at disruptions of human sleep as

reflections of disturbances in a larger, more recently recognized chronobiological "system," the sleep–activity rhythm. A sleep "pacemaker" is thought to exist which coordinates this system. Conveniently enough, it is situated in the brain near input centers from the eyes and the pineal gland, and sits astride pathways from structures deeper within the brain which regulate vegetative functions such as circulation, respiration, and temperature. It is called the suprachiasmatic nucleus and is coordinated in some grand hierarchical, neurological scheme with structures such as the reticular activating system, the thalamus, the hypothalamus, the brainstem structures, and the forebrain, as well as with the multiple different peptides (with names such as neuropeptides, cholecystokinin, and vasoactive intestinal peptide), and with elemental cations such as calcium and magnesium . . . and ultimately ends up using environmental temporal cues (called "Zeitgebers") as well in its overall orchestration of the sleep–wake cycle.

As we have already established, all mammals sleep, although for varying lengths of time. In a general sense, it seems that longer-sleeping animals tend to have shorter lifespans. Whether this is related to excessive amounts of sleep *per se* or, more likely, to some other common denominator perhaps related to metabolic rates, remains to be seen. Although the function and biological meaning of sleep are obscure, sleep does seem to be an important physiological concomitant of processes associated with memory consolidation, body healing, and mood regulation. Certainly we know that in spite of a lack of specific knowledge of the biological purposes of sleep, terrorist torturers and political brainwashers have appreciated the disruptive influence and compelling drive associated with sleep deprivation.

Before going further in our discussion of the relationship between sleep and performance, a number of issues need to be reviewed. These are:

1. the phenomenon of information storage and memory
2. brain laterality
3. distinctions made by behavioral scientists regarding "trait" properties and "state" features, and the circumstance known as "state-dependent learning"
4. thoughts about definitions of "creativity"

Then we can go on to talk about sleep efficiency and some of the nuts-and-bolts issues about the effects of different kinds and qualities of sleep on performance, as well as the effect of certain of life's activities on sleep.

MEMORY AND INFORMATION STORAGE

Like the archives of an august learning institution which allow its members access to systematically stored records of facts and observations, thereby broadening their repertoire, the data-bank of our minds, memory, allows us to broaden the base from which our behavior springs. Internal states which energize behavior impel us toward a particular end. The behavior which emerges is, however, guided by our awareness, analysis, and valuation of both the "driving" internal state and external circumstances surrounding us. "Environment," therefore, takes on a larger meaning, taking into account both the external and the internal milieus. In fact, the internal state of an individual will often affect his perception of external events and may influence the internal processing of stimulus inputs. A well-known example of this is the difference between obese and non-obese people in their responsiveness to food-related stimuli. Obese individuals, as a group, are much more reactive to such cues than are their slimmer counterparts. We will discuss more of this when we turn our attention to state-dependent learning, below.

Memory, therefore, supplies a major dimension to the "environment" in which we operate. Within this databank we store information that helps guide our behavior, sometimes within our conscious ken, oftentimes outside the reaches of consciousness. But in memory we do not store literal recordings of our experience. We store, rather, representations of experience, priority being given in the storage process to representations which have assumed a more exalted place by virtue of the individual's exposure to the experience. For example, depending on an individual's experience with a particular class of objects, the number of models or representations of this particular thing will be determined. Take the example of Eskimos and snow. The Inuktitut language has approximately thirty different words to describe "snow." Incidently, as with any field of knowledge, as more is known, more can be particularized and then, depending on the refinement with which the particular event or object is experienced, the detailed elaboration of the specifics is determined. But remember that these details do not literally represent the "real thing" but only an array of models, probable likenesses derived from different perspectives of the "real thing." The brain is not an unselective pack rat, storing everything experienced. Inputs must have some intensity, some valence associated with them in order to be registered. Then, depending on how our experience elaborates the significance of this information and of those representations already stored, our "memory" will modify the range of the card catalogue display of stored descriptions of classes of experience.

Obtaining some grasp of the function of memory is relevant not only to our understanding of how that functional component of our brain—the mind—works in general, in thought (during both the waking and sleeping states), in action, and in creativity. It will also help us approach understanding the phenomenon of sleep and some of its constituents, like dreams. We are in a remarkably unique situation: I, for instance, am using my mind to describe and understand part of its own experience . . . I think, therefore I am . . . I think!

Memory affects the storage of information, not in the form of literal recordings but, as mentioned before, as representations of classes of objects or experiences. Although our knowledge of how specifically this is accomplished is almost nonexistent, one way that we can look at "information" is to view it as the result of the differential reactivity of neurons in the brain, interwoven in groups or "maps." When these maps then engage each other, "information" results. Whether the memories that chart an individual's history are stored at a biochemical level within particular cells, whether they are held at special storage sites in the brain, in the form of specific anatomic depots, or whether, like the hologram, they are spread throughout the brain in neuronal maps, these traces apparently travel within the brain through a relatively small passageway composed of the brain areas called the temporal lobe of the cortex and the hippocampus. It is not known by what mechanism sensory order is maintained in these archives but it appears, at least from subjective experience, that with sleep, these engrams are released from usual constraints, and memory fragments combine in the formation of dreams.

BRAIN LATERALITY

In the mid 1800s, Paul Broca, a French neurologist, pursued studies of the emplacement and distribution of functions within the brain. He determined that in the majority of people, especially in all righthanded people, the control of functions related to the use of language—that is, speech, reading, and writing—dwells in an area of the **left** cerebral cortex. A neurologist from across the English Channel, John Hughlings Jackson by name, later that century determined that the right cerebral hemisphere was no slouch either when it came to holding administrative sway over important central neurological functions. In this case, the functions pertained to pattern and image recognition—the integration of perceptions, especially those of spatial configurations, as seen by the visual systems of the brain. It then remained for two researchers (Andrew Akelaitis and Roger Sperry) to elaborate upon these findings (work for which Sperry, approximately 25 years later, received the Nobel Prize), to be followed later still by additional work refining previous observations. Thus, a brain "map" denoting the localization of different specialized cognitive functions, was developed, almost like an intracranial phrenology. Additional observations were collected and categorized, tentatively at first, then more certainly as new data were gathered and compared against the initial reference chart. Data were then further collected and collated, the template further edited and revised, and a theory then proposed to further (and more closely) explain the phenomena observed. Such was the process involved in the initial recognition of the "lateralization" of neurological function between the cerebral hemispheres. And such is the process in much of empirical scientific advance: observation, speculation, testing, editing, re-speculation, re-editing . . .

Prior speculation regarding brain function posited a homogeneous and uniform organ with functions bilaterally overlapping and symmetrically distributed between both hemispheres. But assumption of a nervous coupling between the two brain halves notwithstanding, the clinical discovery of a disorder known as alexithymia, which is characterized by difficulty in recognizing and identifying feelings and emotional states (both those of one's own and those of others), helped further support the evolving picture of the distribution of cerebral functions. This discovery also suggested another intriguing tidbit. It suggested a tie-in between cerebral function, creativity and functioning during different behavioral states (especially those associated with the sleep–wake cycle, like dreaming).

It seems that individuals afflicted with alexithymia are excessively literal and unable to exercise imagination and fancy. It is currently assumed that some interference in right hemispheric function accounts for this "pathologic" inability to recognize or process information that we might consider to be "emotional" (as opposed to verbal or logical information, the domain of the left hemisphere). So, we conceptualize each half of the brain, each with its own cognitive specialties resulting in a functional asymmetry between left and right, but intimately interconnected and interactive.

Studies with individuals who, for either surgical or pathological reasons, suffered interference of the band of nerve fibers which runs between the halves of the cortex and provides the interhemispheric highway for transfer of information between both brain halves, led to an appreciation of the so-called "split-brain" phenomenon. "Split-brain" refers to the circumstance in which disruption of the traffic flow between right and left cerebral hemisphere permits information to be presented to only one side of the brain, allowing the individual to act upon this information while having no conscious awareness of this information in the other side of the brain. Then, depending on the mode of information delivery to the individual (that is, whether by words or by images), only one hemisphere would respond. An example: A split-brain individual sits in front of a screen onto which various pictures are projected. He is asked to identify these images. The images are projected in such a way that they fall on that part of the subject's retinae that transmits the perceived images to either the left or the right side of the brain, depending on which the investigator chooses. A picture of a common object, a wallet for instance, is flashed and channeled to the conscious subject's left hemisphere—the seat of his speech center. The subject identifies the object and responds appropriately, verbally. But when the same image is presented to the right hemisphere of the subject, he is not able to respond verbally. He can, however, pick out the correct object by touch from a tray of assorted commonplace objects.

Many varieties and refinements of this experiment have further delineated the nature of the separation of cognitive functions between left and right hemispheres. And what better image?! How neat. Left and right. A clear-cut demarcation of function. Ah, but not so fast. Fond as we may be of dichotomizing into neat categories, be they good guys/bad guys, white hats/black hats, or left brain/right brain (one for speech and the other for everything else), the neurological reality is not so cleanly divided. The bandwagon onto which the popular media and cult-like "how-to" books have recently lept, tends to oversimplify cognitive and neurological function. It reduces complicated mechanisms, systems and phenomena like "creativity" to simple geographical and anatomic "spots," missing totally the subtlety and complexity of underlying neurochemical machinery, while simultaneously underplaying the importance of the coordinated overlap of function and intercommunication between the cerebral hemispheres.

For instance, with regard to "creativity" and the claim that it falls solely under the purview of the right hemisphere, such a position cannot be held any more than can the belief that a specific verbal function, such as reading comprehension, resides solely in the left. Each hemisphere brings different functions to bear in creative tasks, and there is much overlap and perhaps some redundancy of function between the two halves of the cortex. But no creative person who has lost his ability to speak (aphasia), following a left hemispheric stroke, has been able to fully resume prior creative endeavors. Rather than look at these two command centers as independent of each other, we have to look for yet another level of organization to explain the orchestration of cerebral functions.

The archaic view of left cerebral "dominance" has led to several quaint practices such as forcing left-handed children to become right-handed writers or, in the early part of this century, attempting to train that "idle" and "wasted" right brain to take on new functions (shades of which may be seen resurfacing in some of the "self-help" movements of today). The contemporary view is both more complex and less clear: while studies such as those using songbirds have demonstrated the presence of left cerebral dominance with regard to song production, these studies have also shown the presence of the phenomenon of "plasticity" of song production, which implies a relative interchangeability of function between certain central nervous system locations.

Whether a functional and anatomic asymmetry exists, with neurological coupling between hemispheres, each with its own cognitive and perceptual specialty, remains to be seen. Recent studies have suggested that functions previously assigned to either left or right hemispheric locus of action, may in fact alternate, in tides of effectiveness, according to ultradian rhythmic variations. As Gordon and Stoffer pointed out in a series of studies done at the University of Pittsburgh (1989):

> Considerable research effort . . . is spent . . . in quest of an answer to one question: Where, in the brain, are specialized cognitive functions being performed? . . . (But) . . . it is the relative level of ability in **performance** of visuospatial and verbosequential tasks that is important, not the relative activity of the right and left hemispheres during task performance. We propose that brain efficiency for performance of these specialized cognitive tasks is dependent on neurochemical systems rather than on nerve-to-nerve connection or location of specific nerve networks.

With respect to sleep, and in particular to that peculiar form of thinking which occurs during sleep, namely dreaming, let us look at one additional observation of cortical hemispheric functioning, and then turn our attention to a speculation that results from this information. Howard Gardner, at Boston University, has demonstrated that individuals with right-hemispheric brain damage have difficulty understanding the meaning of stories and figures of speech, like metaphor, which use symbolism and substitution of images. They experience a concreteness of thinking, a tendency to focus on and become lost in the literal details, and an inability to see the larger picture—losing the forest for the trees (an image, incidentally, that would not be understandable to you, were you to have sustained this right-hemispheric injury!). It does not seem to be an outrageous speculative leap to assume that, with a shift to the sleeping state (and in particular to the REM sleeping state), the activity level of certain mechanisms regulating aspects of cognition shifts as well. And with this shift, brain focus and attention move from the logical, time-locked detail of daytime thought to a more global neurological perspective in which attention is given to an overall synthesis of both cognitive and emotional inputs. Each state determines a matrix of meaning . . . the waker, a logical narrator, with his daytime discourse; the sleeper, with his dream-poem, more the poet than the essayist.

This descriptive scenario would account for the characteristics of dreams and the cognitive activity called dream-work by psychoanalysts, that we will discuss later in Chapter 8 on dreams. This model of shifting mental states determining the nature of other systems which happen to be functionally coupled, may also account for the apparent parallel between dreams and some of the thinking disturbances present during the waking state in disorders such as schizophrenia. Be it dampened left-hemispheric activity, or heightened right-sided activity, the very nature of thinking shifts from the waking equilibrium established among the neurological functions subserved by the cerebral hemispheres. This shift during the transition from roused state to sleeping state might then account not only for the difference in quality of thinking characteristic of the two states, but also for certain other activities such as sleepwalking or sleep-talking which might follow the release of actions, images, words, or ideas stored in the reservoirs of memory.

STATE-DEPENDENT OBSERVATIONS AND PERFORMANCE

I have introduced the concept of "state dependency" because it has gained increasing popularity among many authors attempting to understand behavioral phenomena. I have further brought it up at this point in an attempt to see if we might utilize our increasing knowledge of the function of the central nervous system, and in particular of the cerebral cortex, in the mediation and control of behavior, to enhance our understanding of aspects of the sleep–wake cycle.

Psychologists use the term "state-dependent learning" (sometimes referred to as "generalization"). Whether we are talking about the neurophysiologist's "state" which by virtue of its very nature allows other behaviors or phenomena to be accessed or to occur (e.g., you can't dance if you're not awake and afoot!), or whether we are referring to a psychological model wherein an accustomed response has been developed to one stimulus and then other similar stimuli will elicit this "conditioned" response, we are talking about the fact that previous experience and status determine the individual's reaction to new situations. These "states" are not the definitive answers in and of themselves; rather, they are phenomena to be explained. As they now stand, they represent descriptive, empirical observations of a class of events or the consequences of a class of events, and are drawn from differing perspectives of different disciplines, watching the same phenomenon. "Explanations" may be in terms of mechanisms or descriptions, whys and hows. So, in one sense, they comprised a type of explanation, since one form of explanation of an event is a comprehensive description of the circumstances under which it occurs, thereby leading to an ability to predict its future occurrence. Of course, however, there are different layers and qualities of description. The question for us, then, in examining various theoretical formulations is "Descriptive at what level?"

The term "state-dependent learning" as often used is incomplete, particularly with regard to mechanisms in which the setting conditions (those conditions which determine the very nature or definition of the particular "state") act. The questions remain, when speaking of "state-dependent" phenomena: What "state" is being referred to? Is it the stimulus property or some other part of the stimulus compound that is assumed to be the operative factor in the particular "state"? Or does a particular "state" refer to a level of arousal? In other words, relying on the phrase "state-dependent" allows authors to avoid coming to grips with what the independent variable really is in the particular situation. They do this by inferring that a "state" exists, rather than that an "effect" has occurred. It would seem that "state-dependent" observations refer to observed changes in the configuration of stimuli that result in particular behaviors (the resultant behaviors would be dubbed "discriminative behaviors" by the experimental psychologist), and as such are really setting conditions, and not just vaguely defined "states."

As an aside, let us briefly take one example of a state-dependent paradigm, as it might be applied to the theory of addictive behavior. State-dependent learning, or stimulus-conditioning theories as we may interchangeably refer to them for our purposes here, view drugs (heroin, marijuana, cocaine, etc.) as modulators of central nervous system and behavior activity. That is, they amplify or inhibit. This modulation then is thought to also influence the perception and processing of contextual factors within which the entire event occurs. The drugged state, then, can serve as a cue and a condition for learning. The intricate hypothesis suggests the following: The state of intoxication (which is the discriminative stimulus and which, once obtained, allows the potential fulfillment of other behaviors that, like a self-perpetuating machine, may then lead to reinforcement in their own right) becomes a conditioned reinforcer, something the addict feels he really wants or needs. Other internal processes might then vary depending upon the level of intoxication, current level of arousal present, and the stages in which the diurnal variation of different humoral agents are. All such factors may function as direct or indirect supporters of an addiction cycle. The above can be used as a paradigm to understand how psychological learning theory can be applied to understanding the modulation of many different activity cycles. We will talk more of this later in the book, when we turn our attention to the disorders of sleeping, and what can be done about them. But for now, let us turn our attention in our discussion of state-dependent phenomena to what is known about the interrelationship between sleep and other behavioral phenomena such as performance and learning.

Various events in our daily existence, from the occurrence of fleeting fantasies and thoughts, to the acquisition of learning, to performance under demand situations, are under the discriminative control of different conditions surrounding the event. What this means, from a psychologist's point of view, is that certain behavioral phenomena can be affected not only by the underlying incentive or motivation, but also by the circumstances around which they occur. We all, whether disciplined student of human behavior or irritated homeowner assessing our neighbor's intention in "letting" his kids cross our newly seeded lawn, try to identify factors responsible for each behavioral event, or portion thereof. And as we do, we come to recognize that factors other than "intention" alone motivate or impel behavior. For instance, stressors of various sorts interact with the sleep–wake cycle to effect insomnia in some. As mentioned before, although the functional meaning of sleep is obscure, it does seem to be an important physiological concomitant to processes such as healing, memory consolidation and mood regulation.

THE STATE/TRAIT DISTINCTION

We now turn our attention to a discussion of the factors which play a role interacting between the physiological (brain) state of sleep and the psychological (mind) state involved in performance and creativity. Whenever the behavioral scientist describes the characteristics of a particular phenomenon, he or she takes into consideration two categories of qualities. One category called a "trait," comprises characteristics such as shyness or extroversion which remain relatively constant over time and through differing circumstances and by which the individual exhibiting them may be more or less consistently recognized. It is from such "personality traits" that we come to predict behavior, assuming that the life circumstances are held constant.

But, of course, life doesn't hold still. The shifting situations of life that form the matrix within which an individual's behavior occurs, form the basis of the second category considered by investigators of behavior. This one is labeled a "state"—a circumstantially determined quality or property. "State" variables change, depending on the conditions and circumstances, and therefore must be studied over time in order to identify dynamic patterns. Further examples of the first group of variables would include heavily biologically determined inclinations such as metabolic activities, intelligence, or certain personality and temperamental features. The second group, that of "state" properties, would include the presence of phenomena such as brief emotional reactions, physical illness, fatigue, or special environmental demands.

To address the questions we all have regarding the interplay between sleep and our efficiency and performance demands that we first answer questions regarding the very qualities of sleep itself. And in order to do that, we must be able to delineate the characteristics of the sleeping state quite clearly. So, with regard to the normal characteristics of sleep architecture, how would one categorize the stages of sleep using the criteria of "trait" and "state"? Or put another way, to what extent is the very structure of sleep relatively fixed and determined for each individual within each species, and to what extent are these structures somewhat malleable in response to shifting circumstantial demands? Furthermore, which aspects of the overall phenomenon of sleep remain relatively consistent over time and circumstance and, therefore, suggest a more fixed, trait-like quality that would be less affected by altering manipulations we might consider employing? And which aspects of sleep, buffeted by the vagaries of day-to-day living, change in response to these demands? Answers to these questions hold importance for anyone seeking to understand sleep disorders and the types of therapeutic interventions that might be effective. So let us try to address some of these inquiries.

For humans, it would seem that total sleep time and the amount of stage 4, NREM sleep are relatively consistent and characteristic for each individual, varying little from night to night, in the absence of outright interference. Such is not true for REM sleep which appears to be, within limits, much more "state"-dependent, as, too, may be the actual timing of the occurrence of the different sleep stages.

What is the evidence that overall sleep time is under the control of a strong, relatively immutable, internal timekeeper? First of all, support for this is found in the numerous examples of the persistence of sleeping even when external conditions, disruptive to well-established time rhythms and schedules, are imposed. If sleep schedules are disrupted or, more drastically, if sleep itself is repeatedly interrupted, the time taken to fall asleep lengthens, the number of awakenings within a sleep cycle increases, and the subjective sense of rest following arousal from the sleep decreases. In other words, "sleep efficiency" of that particular sleep episode declines, while there is an increased pressure to sleep later, in subsequent parts of the individual's sleep—wake cycle. It does seem that a fixed "need" is being disrupted and a "debt" is being accumulated which must, at some point, be satisfied. Secondly, studies involving sudden shifts in work or rest habits, or in day/ night schedules, show that disturbed sleep patterns result, with more frequent arousals within sleep and earlier terminal awakening from sleep, as well as an ensuing reduction in daytime effectiveness. Finally, evidence that sleep seems to be under the control of an internally determined rhythm master is supplied by studies in the sleep laboratory where all time cues (such as natural light, identifying meals, or progressively alternating chores and activities) are removed. When these so-called Zeitgebers (from the German, meaning time-givers) are camouflaged, a daily cycle surfaces which is not our expected 24 hours in length, but one that is 25½ hours long. It is called the "free-running" rhythm.

Although total sleep time and duration of each sleep stage show a striking similarity among comparably-aged people and across different social and cultural contexts, sleep is by no means completely free of the effects of outside factors. Certainly, circumstances as well as individual choice can determine that, at a particular time, sleep will not occur or awakening will. We have just mentioned that, if isolated from time cues such as daylight, clocks, radio and TV, or social interaction with others, we would find ourselves, along with many of our bodily processes including sleep, governed by an inborn, peremptory timekeeping mechanism that even influences how we think at different moments in its cycle. Although the interposition of volitional control is possible (as witnessed by those individuals who can set their conscious alarm clocks in order to "will" themselves awake at a specific hour), the extent to which such basic biological timing machinery can be modified by willingly elected inputs is not yet clear.

And "biological machinery" it is. It remains a challenge and a conundrum for many investigators in the field to attempt to reconcile the data of behavioral "state" with that of biological "state." Let us look for a moment at intriguing findings regarding possible factors involved in the biological regulation of a behavioral state of decreased arousal. If one gathers samples of the liquid medium of the brain (the fluid that bathes the cells of the central nervous system and is rich in proteins, nutrients, and chemicals that help to negotiate the communication from one cell to its neighbor), one can analyze its content and find, suspended within it, molecules that influence behaviors related to temperature control, food intake, and sleep onset. These proteins and polypeptides are the products of the secretory processes of different cells, and change in relation to changes in the metabolism of the secreting cells which, in turn, is affected by (1) variations in cyclical biorhythms, timed by the body's internal clock, and (2) changes in the individual's behavioral state itself.

With regard to this second point, it has been shown that fluid extracts from the brains of sleeping cats contain higher concentrations of certain proteins than in awakened cats, and that samples of this "perfusate" taken from a sleeping cat and introduced into an aroused cat, can induce sleep. So, in a true chicken-and-egg fashion, not only do processes within the central nervous system regulate behavioral states (simultaneously leaving a trail of chemical clues regarding such action), but they are, athwart, themselves, influenced by these very behavioral states! In other words, the level of arousal present at any given moment in the brain, and associated with differing levels of activity, not only is regulated by the basic neuronal structure of the brain, but also regulates, reciprocally, the very neuronal mechanisms underlying functions such as memory, thought, and even elusive phenomena such as creativity and performance.

DETERMINANTS OF PERFORMANCE:
THE ROLE OF SLEEP

In a way, the current chapter, to this point, has served as a preamble to a discussion of the interplay between sleep and performance efficiency, the role of naps, and the interplay among arousal, memory, and imagery in the mental phenomenon we loosely call "creativity." Although the issues are complex and our evolving knowledge far from complete, it is important to place our inquiry regarding puzzling phenomena within a context of information already established. For there is no doubt that the loss of sleep is often experienced by most of us as unpleasant. But it is not clear that this "dysphoria" is related to the loss of sleep itself or to the consequent discoordination of basic biological oscillations. For, much like the kettle's whistle may signal the temperature "state" of the water within, so too might the presence dysphoria blow the whistle on some change or disruption in the underlying biological state. In other words, although alteration of sleep patterns may affect mood and performance, the question remains as to whether this is a direct effect of sleep disruption, or whether sleep disruption is a parallel concomitant to a more significant disruption in any biological rhythm, the results of which are changes in mood and performance. Since any change in the timing and substance of a biological cycle cannot be without effects, the same must be true for sleep. So be it oversleeping, undersleeping, or a shifting of the entire sleep cycle (as with jet lag), this particular change in cycle has effects which must have physiological and behavioral correlates and consequences.

If you have read the newspapers recently, you must have noticed that much has been made of the effect of sleep deprivation on performance, from the overworked hospital intern, to the "yuppie" burning his candle at both ends, to the air traffic controller on the night shift. This is not a new issue, but has risen in prominence in the media. Studies of the effects of one night's sleep deprivation have pointed to various influences on mood and performance which are dependent on factors such as the predeprivation emotional and operational states of the individual, the reason for, and the duration of, the sleep loss. Additionally, much has been made, at times, of the decrement in sleep duration (as well as the prominence of napping) among older adolescents and college students. There are, of course, many circumstances in which general stress factors, social pressures, and the demands of daily living may lead to changes in sleep quality and length. It is important to both recognize these changes and to assess their consequences. But keep in mind that anecdotal and sensationalistic reports of "epidemic" sleep deprivation, coupled with the notoriously unreliable subjective estimates of sleep time, do not necessarily lead to good science or to well-rounded conclusions.

We will talk more of sleep in adolescence later. But for now we turn our attention to real-life examples of sleep deprivation, not just to further delineate the possible functions of sleep, but to assay the effects of different patterns of sleep and of sleep disruption on physical and mental performance in different people under different sets of conditions.

Take doctors, for instance. Recently, much publicity has been given to the suggestion that long work hours, coupled with the attendant sleep loss, have deleterious effects on medical house staff. Certainly bouts of prolonged sleeplessness longer than 24 hours can influence cognitive tasks such as short-term recall and reaction times. But we still function, often because much of our behavior involves responses to already familiar inputs and therefore doesn't demand complex data processing or command functions beyond well-known routines. Evidence also shows that interest and motivation can more than compensate for the effects of sleep deprivation. Furthermore, whenever tested, the individual differences among the different subjects accounted for much more of the difference in task and cognitive performance than did the actual period of sleep deprivation experienced. In fact, it may be that the effect on mood (in terms of irritability, decreased sense of vigor, and increased sense of sadness and social disaffection) may suggest the critical avenue through which sleep deprivation influences performance. Such were findings reported by a colleague of mine, Dr. Richard C. Friedman (1971). It is apparent that such mood changes can magnify effects on the intellectual functioning of selected individuals. But perhaps what more noticeably distinguishes these particular individuals is not who they are but what they are doing. Sleep loss appears to most significantly affect the performance of those who are given uniform, monotonous "vigilance" tasks to carry out in a low-stimulation environment—like long distance drivers, soldiers on watch, or night watchmen at nuclear power plants!

So sleeplessness impairs performance, but its impact can be overcome if the work is interesting or stimulating enough. But what about shift workers . . . individuals constantly placed in schedule changes that lead to circadian rhythm disruptions? When one compares day workers with shift workers (morning or evening) with permanent night workers, one finds that the last category includes people who nap more frequently than their day- or shift-time compatriots. This seems to occur because their day sleep is, on average, shorter in duration than "normal" night sleep.

So some compensatory sleep seems necessary for permanent night workers. But, if they are able to get it, this group reports the fewest tiredness and headache complaints of the three groups. We know instinctively that we "need" to sleep. We do not, however, know how this need may be most efficiently satisfied. Some sleep right through the night, in one prolonged bout of oblivious somnolence. But some shift workers sleep in multiple bouts each 24-hour cycle, and college students are notorious nappers (with estimates in some samples suggesting that 80 percent of college students take frequent naps).

NAPS

It seems that we human beings need at least half of our usual nighttime sleep to fend off slumps in performance during urgent endurance bouts of labor. Therefore, it should not come as a surprise that a nap, no matter how brief, under circumstances of demand and deprivation, may remedy the sense of sleepiness. Whether we are talking of the catnaps of Thomas Edison and Winston Churchill, the late afternoon naps in the far reaches of northern Scandinavia, the tropical siesta, or the middle European *Mittagschlafchen*, napping is a pervasive, but not universal phenomenon. Thirty to 40 percent of Americans rarely, if ever, nap. Most afternoon naps last between 30 and 90 minutes, comprise the deepest, stage 4, sleep with little dreaming, and are often followed by groggy, disoriented "sleep inertia," suggesting that, for many, it is best to get up gradually from a nap.

Napping seems to be an attempt to compensate for the shortening of what would be considered the primary period of sleep. The subjective sense of having had a "good night's sleep" seems correlated with prolonged time spent in one's main period of sleep as well as with a longer duration of total sleep. This, coupled with the fact that what seems to be consistent for each individual is the total sleep time characteristic for him or her, may account for the observation that the major nighttime sleep segment of habitual nappers is shorter than that of nonnappers, but overall, both groups generally sleep comparable amounts of time.

Perhaps because it intervenes as an island of refreshment in a sea of sleepiness that a nap's rejuvenating properties appear exaggerated when compared with the longer duration of the regular sleep episode. Since naps do seem to serve some sort of compensatory or replacement role in the face of general sleep deprivation, probably a nap of any length is better than none at all. But researchers at the Institute of the Pennsylvania Hospital found that a 4-hour nap does not compare in beneficial effects to 8 hours of sleep. In a study published in 1987, Dinges and co-workers tried to determine what would be the best timing for a nap to achieve the maximum salutary effects with regard to alertness and reaction time. They found that napping, in anticipation of a night of sleep loss, can help an individual stand up to the following claims for performance. Furthermore, they found that the absolute presence of any such nap is more important than the specific timing of its occurrence. In fact, there may be a differential effect: napping in anticipation of sleep loss may have positive effects on subsequent actions, while napping during sleep loss may have an effect only on the sense of sleepiness and not on the performance consequences of the sleep loss. It would seem that naps, when taken close enough to the anticipated time of deprivation, can be put "in the bank," to be drawn upon when sleep loss does in fact occur. But making such deposits when the bank is already in deficit, although it may lead the depositor to feel somewhat more flush, has little substantive use when subsequent performance demands require a mobilization of resources!

Although the aftereffects of naps on performance and the subjective sense of well-being remain to be systematically investigated, they do seem to depend on the timing of the nap (and on whether the nap is taken during the heights or the lows of underlying circadian alertness cycles) and the types of measurements used. Even at this early stage in our knowledge, one finding does seem clear. For those who nap without sleep loss but just as a habitual part of their normal sleep cycle, the nap's effect on their mood is considerably more marked than its actual effect on their performance (as measured by changes in reaction time). Naps do improve mood in people who like to nap and who do it frequently. But people who do not seek out naps nor nap frequently often feel soured after one. Even with this observation, there are confounding considerations.

There are two findings which can muddy the waters regarding any conclusion about the benefits of napping on performance. First, there is the phenomenon known as "sleep inertia"—that logy, fuzzy feeling one often experiences immediately upon arising from a nap. This short-lived post-awakening reduction in performance will affect any measure of activity (and, in fact, may occur in another, less abbreviated form following morning rising, leading to the rush for the shower and the coffee pot). Second, in experimental subjects, just the knowledge that a rest break is coming from the laboratory's sleep-loss protocol leads to improved cognitive performance. In fact, Dr. Martin Orne has spent much of his professional life elegantly delineating, in a controlled, laboratory setting, the extent to which expectation and anticipation color the experience of an event and even determine motivation and outcome in studies of human behavioral phenomena like sleep and hypnosis. Finally, it is not at all clear that the nap, and its attendant sleep, are the critical factors in mood alterations (like decrease in feelings of anxiety and confusion and reduction in a sense of fatigue), or whether (1) other more profound and intricately interwoven biorhythmic effects, or (2) just the occasion of resting in bed, which nap behavior provides, is the crucial factor.

Whether naps serve to ameliorate a sense of sleepiness, whether they in fact help in mood and cognitive recovery from sleep loss, or whether they have effects combining both aspects of mental life in varying degrees depending on the timing and conditions under which a nap is taken, we are on the threshold of answering these questions. In the meantime, we know that naps often leave us feeling less exhausted, but not until several post-awakening minutes have elapsed. We also know that nappers, as opposed to nonnappers, seem to be in more conscious control of the ability to fall asleep. If we were to divide all people into three groups according to their napping habits ("habitual nappers," "replacement nappers," and "nonnappers"), we would know that all three groups show no REM sleep during naps and all demonstrate similar 24-hour total sleep time. What does differ among them is the sleep architecture, with the habitual nappers demonstrating much more fluctuation among sleep stages during their main sleep period, and a predominance of stage 1 sleep during the nap.

Naps, like sleep, like most behavioral phenomena, are not unitary, monolithic events. They can serve to satisfy functions ranging from the physiological to the psychological, and allow for broad ranges in individual differences in dimensions and traits. They can allow for a number of different underlying mechanisms to affect them, and can provide a final common pathway for the expression of behavior whose underpinnings may have originated from various and diverse sources.

Chapter 5

The Early Bird Catches the Worm, so Let Me Sleep on It
Sleepiness, Performance, and Creativity

SLEEPINESS AND NAPS

It has been said that life imitates art. Well, perhaps. But in a case just recently reported, life, it seems, imitates the artist, or at least the legend of an artist: Leonardo da Vinci, driven by his need to make time for his many pursuits in the arts and science, is rumored to have slept only one and one-half hours a day . . . this, by taking 15-minute catnaps every four hours.

In a recent study noted in the journal *Science*, a researcher by the name of Claudio Stampi was able to place a 27-year-old volunteer on a "sleep diet," averaging 2.7 hours of sleep a day, by scheduling repetitive cycles of six 15-minute naps daily. Although there was no evidence of any decrement in performance over a 9-day period, the longer-term consequences of such a regimen have not been determined (with respect either to enhanced productivity or to possible detrimental complications). Stampi did, however, note a possible confounding issue: if you are able to free up all that extra time by sleeping less, you will have to know what to do with it!

We are just beginning to understand that the sense of daytime sleepiness (a complaint which many have and which many feel interferes with the productivity of their daily lives) may, in some, be related to repeated mini-episodes of nighttime electrical showers in the brain that increase muscle tone and, although insufficient to lead to full-fledged awakening, are sufficient to fragment the normal sleep architecture. These arousals-without-awakenings, in addition to other disruptive influences on the sleep cycle's coherence (like advancing age, various medical conditions, work shift demands, and jet lag), have led researchers to look to naps and their reputed restorative effects for possible insights into the recuperative effects of sleep in general.

If sleep does function in order to soothe, we have not yet identified the "toxin" produced by the waking or aroused brain for which sleep is the counteractant. In this search, sleep investigators have turned their attention to stage 4 (or "slow wave" or "delta") sleep because the amount of stage 4 sleep appears to be directly related to the duration of presleep awake time and yet remains at constant levels with partial sleep deprivation. That is, other sleep stages are sacrificed but not stage 4. In addition, stage 4 sleep recedes as the night progresses, as if it is drained as some store is being replenished or, alternatively, as some residual by-product of the preceding waking state is being disposed of and neutralized.

Another dimension that researchers monitor in their quest for understanding the function of sleep is the effect of sleep loss on performance, be it physical or mental. Here one can subject a person to a fixed amount of work and see how his capacity to do this work changes with increasing sleep deprivation and recovery from bouts of sleep loss. From such studies, results regarding muscular work suggest that there is little if any change in the capacity to do aerobic muscular work following partial sleep deprivation. Any fall-off in actual muscular performance or en-durance seems more related to changes in psychological factors. (But the subjects do yawn more! And this yawning does, in such experimental circumstances, seem to be responsive to factors beyond just the psychological. Although the meaning of yawning has not been established, it is one more phenomenon in a series of observations, which suggests that respiratory regulation is sensitive to alterations in levels of arousal.)

Metabolic changes do occur with prolonged sleep deprivation, however. These include a decrease in one's resting body temperature and, for many, an increase in hunger. Both of these further support the interweaving of sleep-regulatory and metabolic and temperature-regulatory mechanisms discussed earlier. But as with all observed changes that occur with sleep loss, the question must be answered as to whether these alterations are related to the sleep loss per se or are rather consequent to the stress associated with a bout of sleep loss. And even more than "stress," the relevant consideration may be the presence of "distress." For all life is filled with challenge, with obstacles to be overcome, with situations to be mastered . . . with stress.

The significant differential consideration is not necessarily whether or not "stress" exists, but whether or not concomitant apprehension or psychological "distress" exists. It is this latter phenomenon which can further impact on central nervous system mechanisms that may ultimately affect (as well as be affected by) central biological rhythmic processes. So, when claims are made that a person's immune response, for instance, is depressed with sleep loss, thereby making him more susceptible to illness, it remains to be seen whether it is the sleep loss itself that is the causative factor (and that sleep replenishment should be considered the primary ameliorative factor), or whether attention to the alleviation of stress might be the more prudent focus of therapeutic effort.

We spoke, in the previous chapter, about naps as possible clues to a restorative, or at least a deficit-replacement, function for sleep. For, unlike the Federal Government, the Sleep Bureaucracy will not hold on to a deficit budget for long. In this regard, there has been some public concern recently expressed over the long work hours of young doctors-in-training, and the possible effects of sleep deprivation on their hospital performance. An outcry has led to a number of state legislatures passing bills restricting the number of continuous hours that hospital house staff can be required to work. However, we are not talking about restrictions to an 8-hour work day! The average hospital intern works considerably longer hours than that and is still required to tend to his or her emergency patients through prolonged stints. We saw from our discussion in the previous chapter that perhaps it would have made more sense for hospital administrators to provide nap time for their overworked interns. Instead, legislators, with incomplete knowledge of the phenomenon involved and yielding to public pressure, demanded minimal reductions in work hours which still permit the unrelieved presence of prolonged periods of sleep deprivation of up to 48 hours.

And what about college students who must curtail some of their sleep time for cramming time? Which is better for performance: staying up later while keeping the same rising time, or getting more sleep and then waking early to put the cramming-icing on the studying-cake? Well, allowing for individual differences in vigilance and clear-wittedness, as well as variations in certain physiological parameters such as body temperature and individual differences in mood, motivation, and reaction time, early rising is more disruptive for more people than is postponed bedtime. If, in addition, the person is a "night person" or has been up for several nights with an accumulating amount of sleep loss, the disruption will be magnified. (And, yes, Virginia, there are "night" and "morning" people . . . the former always having difficulty rising early in the morning. Also, Virginia, although this may be related to subtle shifts in individual circadian rhythm traits, it may alternatively be related to characteristic differences in the metabolic substrate that determines post-sleep inertia.)

So, if you are a "night person" who can procrastinate no longer and **must** study for this exam, chances are you'd be better off burning the midnight oil rather than being the early bird. Because if you are referring to increased performance following early morning awakening, for most people it is probably **not** true that the early bird catches the worm.

SLEEP AND PERFORMANCE

In assessing the effects of sleep on modes of thinking, on aspects of physiological functioning, and, therefore, on performance, it is always difficult to test, to dissect out, the influence and contribution of factors such as interest and motivation. For instance, with complex undertakings such as decision-making or reading comprehension, sleep deprivation does not seem to have an immediate effect on the accomplishment of these tasks because of the compensatory effects of the stimulating demand of the work itself—a stimulation that apparently compensates more than enough for any sleepiness-induced falloff in desire. However, there is another form of cognition, the activity associated with creative thinking, which involves qualities and skills such as originality, spontaneity of thinking, and flexibility and adaptability of response, which does seem to be more influenced by sleep deprivation when tested in experimental subjects. To what extent this is due to a falloff in motivation and interest consequent to sleep loss, and to what extent it is secondary to a sleep loss-induced decrease in ability to think in this particular mode are not yet clear. No doubt both may apply.

It is inevitable that we will question the role of sleep (and dreams) in processes related to creative acts. The reasoning draws from topics reviewed in the previous chapter, and goes as follows: The interplay between both "trait" and "state" qualities determines the extent of creativity present in any given individual; prerequisites for creative endeavors include access to stores of prior experience and training (memory), an ease with the control of the borderline between fantasy thinking and reality thinking, and an ability to travel between linear, logical thinking and more spatial, global impressionistic thought processes with facility (left brain/right brain); an ability to permit internal representations or images of the mind to gestate, coupled with a plasticity of certain processes (like memory consolidation) responsive to behavioral state influences (state-dependency) are, additionally, important foundations for the creative process.

With regard to this last point, "sleep" is of interest when we turn our attention to the influence of different behavioral levels of arousal on both psychological and physiological functioning underlying the creative process. Since different neuronal cell activities vary and correlate with specific levels of central nervous system arousal, from waking to sleeping, the question arises whether subtle differences in behavioral states of arousal allow differential access to variants of creative thinking and result in different performance potentials within the same individual at different times. Such an interdependence may be likened to the priming of a pump, wherein the particular level of behavioral activation serves as the prime for the correlative psychological and physiological functions.

Let us return to an earlier analogy of the tidal rhythms. Our very biological and psychological existence is composed of an interlocking multilayered orchestration of monthly, daily, and hourly rhythms, some becoming more apparent only as others temporarily recede to reveal the pulsations underneath. We might liken the situation of larger, overriding rhythms masking underlying ones, to the pattern of the ebbing and flowing daily tide which covers, but periodically reveals, the more microscopic rhythms of crustacean life in the tidal pools below that proceed regardless of the larger, masking, concurrent rhythm. Perhaps this same characterization may be applied to an ongoing ultradian rhythm relentlessly pulsing but masked beneath its larger, circadian cousins. Some investigators assume that the NREM–REM sleep cycle continues throughout the day, oscillating along with different phases of the circadian rest/activity cycle. And it is only when the larger circadian cycle swings through its nadir of inactivity, during sleep, that the NREM–REM cycle stands out in bolder relief and appears more evident. Such varying interrelationships as these, among different biological processes, then, define different "states" of the individual. And these different neuronally determined states, along with their adjunctive behavioral components, influence other aspects of physiological functioning, such as circulation, breathing, and temperature regulation.

Of course, life is a two-way street, and complexly interwoven systems affect, as well as are affected by, each other. The yogi practicing breath control can affect his level of arousal (his conscious state, if you will) just as much as his transition from the neuronal activity of wakefulness to that of sleep will affect the regulation of his breathing. The same presumably is true for other metabolic and physiologic areas.

We intuitively understand this concept when considering the hyperexcitable "Type A" dynamo and his blood pressure. And if relationships exist between behavioral states like the sleep–wake cycle and specific organ systems, we have the potential for investigating the involvement of these cycles in different psychological phenomena and in various pathological states (like the Sudden

Infant Death Syndrome, or nighttime heart attacks). As one, brief, tantalizing example: we have talked about the important role of the neurotransmitter serotonin in the regulation of the sleep–wake cycle, and we will discuss it more in Chapter 6. For now, let us further note that serotonin has been implicated as:

1. an important factor in the regulation of mood
2. an important central nervous system facilitator of respiration control
3. a key player in nerve cells in the part of the central nervous system, called the hypothalamus, which regulate body temperature
4. a component of other central nervous system neurons regulating the cardiovascular system
5. an activator of disease-fighting "macrophage cells" in the immune system (an action it shares with what is considered by some to be a naturally occurring, sleep-promoting substance called muramyl peptide)

Here is but one example of a matrix in which not only can physiology affect the "state" of the organism, but in which the state can also affect physiology, by complex and confounding feedback, all tied together by a neurochemical common denominator.

In our discussion of the interaction between "states" and concomitant behavioral/physiological processes, let us now turn our attention more specifically to the effects of sleep deprivation on performance. To re-emphasize: Uncomplicated, unchallenging, repetitive or monotonous, and prolonged tasks are the ones most influenced by sleep deprivation. Under these circumstances, effects such as decreased ability to concentrate, the experiencing of visual distortions and illusions, irritability and increased suggestibility, as well as, of course, an increased sense of sleepiness—can all be experienced. And **all** can be ameliorated, at least to some extent, by the application of incentives, by increasing the inherent interest and challenge of the required task, or by superimposing the natural increase in arousal which occurs during the early daytime portion of the circadian rhythm . . . remember our discussion earlier of the interdigitation and layering of cycles and the masking of the effects of one cycle by a more prominent, coexisting one.

It should be noted that most of the troublesome and untoward effects of sleep deprivation on behavior and performance are corrected after only one night of sleep recovery. And, interestingly, it is not necessary for the total amount of recovery sleep to replace, on a one-for-one basis, the number of hours lost, for full improvement in performance to occur. This observation has led prominent sleep researcher J. A. Horne (1988) to hypothesize that only the first 4–6 hours of a normal night's sleep (that is, the segment which contains the major portion of stage 4 sleep) is necessary for the maintenance of a normal state of health. This, Horne calls "obligatory sleep," leaving the last hours of sleep as "facultative," as icing on the sleep-cycle cake, the loss of which does not affect daytime sleepiness. According to Horne, the "facultative" component of sleep varies in response to environmental factors such as stress, distractions, and challenge. And, in fact, a study of people who have had chronic insomnia for many years, reportedly unable ever to sleep for more than 5 hours any night, showed no differences in performance when tested and compared with sleepers getting what would be considered to be a full complement of nightly rest on a regular basis.

The situation is somewhat different, however, for those individuals who, because of environmental disturbances or certain medical and sleep-related disorders, suffer brief regularly recurring episodes of interruption throughout the sleep cycle, with consequent daytime sleepiness and performance falloff. Here, the effects of sleep loss, based on brief disruptive stimuli to which the sleeper adapts and therefore never fully experiences consciously, are just as prominent as in situations where a person is forceably kept awake. And in both circumstances, the sleep-deprived individual will demonstrate a typical repercussive increase in sleep if permitted . . . the so-called sleep "rebound."

Having read this far, therefore, and faced with the latest health-fad media blitz highlighting dramatic claims that we are all sleep-deprived, you are now far better able to explore the issue, evaluate the warning, and test for the presence of such a phenomenon. We do not have to fall into lockstep and, with nimble but uncritical footwork, jump onto this bandwagon unnecessarily. We can even save a little money by not buying the latest book claiming to offer a self-help remedy for a possibly nonexistent malady.

And how are we to accomplish this? By addressing four issues: First, when confronting such a claim, we must ask, what does "sleep deprived" mean? We know that individuals have changing needs for sleep, which also vary depending on differing demands and different times of their lives. So a so-called normative **number** really does not exist, although a normative **range** might.

Second, we must ask, what is the manifestation of such deprivation? Daytime sleepiness? Performance lapses? Decreased time in bed is certainly a critical factor in determining the presence of daytime sleepiness. (Incidentally, as such a determinant, time in bed far outweighs in importance either the effects of alcohol or of caffeine in a well-rested person. In other words, the next-day effects of alcohol, or the same-day effects of caffeine on daytime sleepiness are relatively minimal, compared with actual loss of bed time.) There are, of course, other causes of daytime sleepiness, like certain long-acting tranquilizers or some antihistamines taken at bedtime. Therefore, daytime sleepiness alone cannot be used as a sole criterion for the presence of sleep deprivation.

Third, physical activity affects the duration of sleep, and, in particular, the architecture of the sleep cycle. REM sleep is shortened in physically fit individuals, but this may be more related to the connection between energy expenditure and REM cycles in those people with higher metabolic rates. It has also been reported that, following exercise, there is an increase in stage 4, NREM sleep (questions about the significance of which we have previously discussed). These changes too, however, are associated with alterations in brain temperature (and no direct effect on muscle restitution has yet been demonstrated). Furthermore, there are those who point out that an established state of physical fitness (as opposed to an acute bout of exercise) is not associated with any particularly notable pattern of sleep duration nor with the particular prominence of stage 4 sleep. So one must evaluate concerns about sleep "deprivation" in light of recent changes in physical activity level as well.

Finally, the fourth issue: We know that sleep-deprived individuals, if given the opportunity to catch up for lost sleep, will indeed do so. They will experience a sleep rebound. Consequently, and barring any unusual circumstance, if you are concerned that you have, in the rush and hub-bub of a high pressured existence, created a sleep-deprived record for yourself, test it. Allow yourself some uninterrupted sleep time to determine whether your internal clock will attempt to make up for lost time if given the chance. And if you are such a driven person that you cannot permit yourself such a "luxury," perhaps calling it a "test" will help!

SLEEP AND CREATIVITY

Let us assume there are two "blind men," one a so-called "hard science" biologist, the other a so-called "soft science" psychoanalyst, both examining the same sleeping individual, or so-called "elephant." They are asked, does the activity going on within the sleeper's mind (or "brain") have intent? Unfortunately, too often they each look at the indirect indicators of mentation during sleep (such as squiggles on the EEG record or dream reports) only from their own biased but similarly limited, mono-dimensional perspective, and reach arbitrary, mutually exclusive, but insistent conclusions. The psychoanalyst says, "Why yes, of course the sleeping mind has intent and its productions have meaning!" and then goes on to concoct an intricate metapsychology to "explain" his conclusion. The biologist, just as definitively from his vantage point says, "No, the productions of the sleeping brain are merely the equivalents of biological noise!" and proceeds to blindly dismiss the reality of psychological "meaning" in human existence and to discard the validity and applicability of inputs from other disciplines. Let us try to correct such shortsightedness, and, by considering these complex phenomena from a number of different perspectives, flesh out the bones of more meager, uni-dimensional, and parochial perspectives.

It would seem that one's cognitive activity (or thought processing, if you will) not only varies between waking and sleeping states, but also changes within sleeping life, differing in quality depending on whether one is in a REM or a NREM stage of repose. Let us, for the sake of argument, conceive of the brain as a cognitive, tale-spinning machine in perpetual motion, generating a constant flow of thoughts and images, interlinking data taken in with that already stored, and further scanning and modifying this store of information with each new intrusion of external stimuli.

This brain sleeps in both REM and NREM stages. With REM sleep there is an increasing activity of the brain's cortical neurons, whose behavior then resembles that of the fully awake state. Additionally, there is a heightened barrier to the intrusion of external, "distracting" inputs. It had initially been hypothesized that this reciprocal relationship between increased cognitive activity and reduced responsiveness to external stimuli served some functional purpose, perhaps reflecting the brain's reworking ad consolidation of the previous day's data within its larger memory reservoir.

The fact that REM sleep may play a role in the memory process has been suggested for some time. For instance, the eventual mastery and completion of complex learning tasks seemed to result in increased amounts of REM sleep. Furthermore, if laboratory animals were selectively deprived of REM sleep, they showed impaired retention of acquired learning in complex-task situations. As a result, some have hypothesized that an aspect of generalized brain activation (like the kind that occurs during REM sleep) is crucial to the memory coalescing process. Just like the pregame pep talk heightens a team's "energy" level and, presumably, has a favorable impact on their subsequent performance, so too might the particular REM state of arousal (without the distraction of awakening) serve to facilitate reworking the constant flow of data bits and pieces which, when integrated, will solidify into memory.

In an attempt to further delineate the kind of thinking that may go on during sleep, several recent studies have successfully presented sound cues, during REM sleep, to sleepers who had just learned a task that demanded auditory attention. By matching the cue to the particular sensory modality used during the learning, the researchers were in fact able to enhance the learning. From this, and other studies as well, it follows that sleeping individuals are clearly able to "perceive" certain inputs and can muster some response to them, even though asleep. Obviously, therefore, some sort of assessment and analysis is going on. But does this mean that learning is possible during sleep?

It is known that, with appropriate presleep training, sleepers can respond to certain stimuli presented to them during sleep. Although the level of responsiveness to such external cues is much less than what occurs during waking, evidence of "awareness" to stimulus factors, both externally delivered and internally generated, is definitely present. However, it is only in stage 1, NREM sleep, in that lightest of sleep stages, when it is often difficult to tell whether a person is slightly asleep or barely awake, that the learning of externally presented material seems at all possible.

With regard to the retention of material that has been recently learned, this preservation is often improved when the learning period is followed by some sleep time. It is also known that simple behaviors learned in the researcher's laboratory (like the control of one's breathing rhythms) can be affected by subtle, nondisruptive stimuli given during sleep. Yet, however intriguing the suggestions are regarding the ability to register and incorporate inputs that are presented to us "subliminally" (that is, outside of our conscious awareness, whether asleep or awake), we still remain unable to definitely account for any such phenomena. Since, by definition, we are referring to a cognitive process which, although it demands no conscious attention, does have an impact on a person's conscious thoughts and actions, we are really questioning whether an individual can, purposely and with intention, process information of which he is not consciously aware!

A brief aside: We take for granted that our brains "work." But in a fit of blind "inattention," perhaps coupled with an "arrogance of consciousness," we not only can be dismissive of that part of our experience which involves interlaced levels of information stored outside of our conscious awareness; we can go so far as to deny, outright, its very existence. We do this despite the fact that the very occurrence of the phenomenon of dreaming, taking place as it does during a state of reduced consciousness, is a testimonial to the presence of system involved in at least the partial retrieval of remembrances stored from previous experiences. We can also deny the impact of unconscious processes on our conscious lives even though we know that an individual is only able to respond to a small portion of the input information presented to him at any given instant. It **must** be possible for the information-processing apparatus of the brain to perform triage . . . to select, on a priority basis, which signals will be attended to, which will be stored as part of the gallery-of-memory's "permanent" collection, and which will be momentarily put aside in storage, for subsequent consideration and processing, once disposition of those inputs felt to have more urgency has been done.

It is not a far leap from an appreciation of this intricacy of the attention/information-processing/memory systems that stand between our experience and the complex world about us, to the hypothesis that part of the work of sleep is intimately connected with the operation of these systems, allowing the encoding of data and the translation of inputs into memory. As we will discuss in Chapter 7, different theorists propose different ways that REM sleep, and its epiphenomenon, dreaming, might serve the function of consolidating inputs into memory stores and then might maintain them. An example is the proposal of Crick and Mitchison in 1983 (the first of whom you may recognize as one of the Nobel Prize winners for the discovery of the structure of that core genetic material DNA). They suggest that REM sleep serves a housekeeping function during which the "chaff" of the day's memory traces is separated from the "wheat" of the retained memories. In the process, extraneous noise and unnecessary data are edited out. They, incidentally, use as "evidence" for such an information-forgetting function of sleep and dreams the very fact that dreams are forgotten. In other words, according to Crick and Mitchison, we dream in order to forget, thereby allowing a less-encumbered brain to function more efficiently.

Of course, Sigmund Freud proposed an entirely different mechanism. To foreshadow our discussion of Chapter 8, Freud felt that the purpose of dreaming (at least in part) was to help maintain the sleeping state, to shield the sleeper from the disruptive effects of extraneous stimuli. This, he proposed, was accomplished by incorporating potentially disturbing stimulus events into the ongoing flow of the sleep mental activity. That is, disruptive inputs would be absorbed into, and neutralized by, the matrix of the sleeper's dreaming. Whether or not a "mechanism" of mental incorporation, or one of mental housecleaning, or some combination of both really are factors, remains to be established. It furthermore remains to be seen whether these hypotheses reflect "functions" or "purposes" of dreaming, or whether dreaming is but a correlative concomitant of the mental shutdown to external events that occurs during sleep, where attention to the world of external stimuli is dampened. For "attention" (or "conscious awareness") may serve as a telescope which is turned toward a particular target. In this somewhat incompletely wrought analogy, as one zooms in on the target, one focuses on that object.

However, if there is no external object, and without the "distraction" of that distant object of interest, one may become aware instead of the very presence and functioning of the telescope itself. In a similar fashion, perhaps REM sleep, like sensory deprivation or trance-like dissociative states, allows the redirection and inward focusing of the mind's eye onto a continuous associative flow of internal mind/brain events.

To return to our discussion of subliminal phenomena: What we do know is that a critical factor, which determines whether an individual will "attend" to a particular input, is what we might loosely call the "salience" of that particular stimulus for the particular individual receiving it. The advertising message visually embedded in the TV picture, flashed on the screen at speeds fast enough to be below the threshold of conscious perception, will affect the viewer only under very special and limited conditions. In the case of a subliminal advertisement urging the consumption of a particular brand of soda, for instance, these conditions would include the following: the specific presence of thirst and the intention to slake it; the easy accessibility to an immediate source of the commodity so that the short-lived effects of the suggestion can be acted upon before they rapidly dissipate; and the presence of plainness, directness, and simplicity in the message itself.

For those of us who try to understand the processes by which mental effects are interconnected and interact, we must not lose sight of the slippery issue which we called "salience" above, and which also goes by the name "meaning." Take, for example, the interrelationships among sleep, performance, and creativity: It is all well and good to perform a study by presenting a subject with a presleep stimulus and instructing him how to respond to it, then allowing him to sleep and presenting the signal to him at various times during his sleep cycle. You may then assay:

1. his responsiveness to the stimulus, at different REM and NREM sleep times
2. changes in his sleep architecture and timing
3. signs of possible incorporation of this signal into his sleep mentation, that is, into his dreams

But meanings can be transformed and interchanged, and what is incorporated may be a symbolic analogue which is idiosyncratic to the particular subject and whose significance, therefore, is not recognized by the particular researchers. So, although there does seem to be a relationship between sleep mental activity and reactivity to external stimulation, the hope to passively learn specific and complex tasks, administered to us while we sleep, is but a pipe dream. Our magical wish for an easy way to learn French notwithstanding, the heightened barrier to external sensory inputs that occurs during sleep is a fact, and a fact which probably reveals something about the natural activity of our brain's mind. When not commanded by some peremptory external stimulus, our minds can wander; we can daydream. And when put in an isolation tank, devoid of any sensory stimulation, our minds can hallucinate, as if undistracted by the intermittent intrusions of the external world which had been carried to us through our senses.

Why not, then, assume, as some researchers have, that since we perform constant mental activity, whether asleep or awake, perhaps some purpose to this activity can be expected even when asleep. For instance, in order to remember things while awake, we oftentimes rehearse them. We use a piece of information, a skill, over and over, and it becomes more comfortable and an easier part of our regular repertoire. And with disuse, we seem to lose the facility with, and the accessibility to, certain bits of information, be they recollections or skills. It is an extension of this commonplace experience that led some to postulate that, if daytime experiential and sensory inputs are to be incorporated into our data reservoir for future use, they must be exercised and reinforced. This assumption really explains little with regard to how the processes of sleeping and dreaming might accomplish this incorporation and consolidation of information accumulated by the individual during his waking hours, but it suggests a beginning theoretical framework . . . but only a beginning.

Further lacking is any understanding of how the information that is retained is stored, or how, for that matter, this particular information is selected out of all data that have impressed themselves upon the individual during the previous day. Perhaps the enormity of the explanatory task led investigators like Crick and Mitchison to turn away from the intricacies of memory mechanisms, to focus instead on housekeeping and editing functions. It is here, although at a different level of discourse, that Freudian notions, regarding the role that emotions play in the selection process which brings information bits into memory stores and maintains them there, attempted to reconcile mechanistic theories, both psychological and biological, about the function of sleep and dreams with respect to learning, performance, and creativity.

For many who wrestle with creative endeavors—be they painter, poet, landscape designer, or the virtuoso traffic cop, speeding us through a potentially grid-locked intersection with balletic grace—the sole element of creativity does not necessarily rest with finding just the right element, but rather, in working and reworking the different elements to produce a coherent sensorily objective embodiment (the created product) of a state of mind or vision. From this point of view, the larger issue is constructing the right composition from the different available and selected components in order to create an event, an effect, rather than a particular object (the latter might be viewed more as a "craft" than as a creative work of "art," but that distinction is probably a little too fine for our discussion about creativity here). The object created, in turn, abundant in transposed symbolic designation and metaphor, embodies this effect or state of mind.

As discussed before, most likely a sizeable portion of our mental activity comes to pass outside of our conscious awareness. As any of us will recognize, our attention has a rather narrow range and, at any particular instant, is focused only on small parts of the entire flow of inputs cascading onto our various sensory channels. For instance, until I mention it, you are not attentive to . . . the bottoms of your feet! But, once called to your attention, you instantly know their location and condition. Some monitoring, outside of your conscious attention had, no doubt, been going on and, had the need arisen, you would have quickly incorporated that information into some behavioral matrix and brought it to consciousness, facilitated either by some external urgency or by some peremptory, inner "somesthetic" cue.

Since, again, the process of attention is finite in its scope, only a small portion of our total sensory experience can be focused on at any particular moment. Obviously, then, a certain amount, perhaps a large amount, of input escapes attention and does not enter into the subjective experience of "awareness." However, even though they are "unconscious," these inputs are essential determinants of some aspects of our cognitive, emotional and motivated behaviors.

Imagine, if you will, that the difference between conscious and unconscious experience is the length of time that particular cells in the brain's cerebral cortex are activated. Turn the switch on and brain circuits quicken, and the individual experiences the neuronal machinations as manifestations of consciousness. But just briefly throw the switch, or turn the power on so low that subthreshold amounts of brain circuit activation result, and you end up with neuronal functioning on an unconscious basis. This distinction is raised when we consider phenomena such as subliminal stimulation and "perception," "free will," and choice-making, or the creative and "intuitive" thinking process of the artist, the scientist, and the inventor. Future investigation will attempt to understand the mental and physiological states that may affect the focus of attention and may also permit access to other arenas of mental activity that have eluded the daytime, waking eye of attention processes. And it is within this context that further clarification of issues such as the effect of differing states of sleep and arousal on learning, performance efficiency, and creativity will be found.

We are not the first to be intrigued by the interplay between internal representations, or images of the mind, and memory, for example. The ancient Greeks used imagery in exercises meant to promote and enhance memory. We are not the first to speculate about differing "mind states," the mind's use of images and the creative process. The scientist Kekule dreamt of a ring of snakes and, reportedly, from this remembered image discovered the molecular structure of the benzene ring . . . a key component of the pervasive element, carbon. And we are not the first to assume the importance (if not primacy) of visual or pictorial representation in the undergirding of cognition, nor the first to point to the significance of this form of mental representation and the role it might play in establishing the power of metaphor within the "language of thought."

It has become clear in experimental studies that visual experience, during critical developmental periods, affects the development of the visual system within the brain . . . even down to determining characteristics of the connections among nerve cells within that system. This plasticity, as it is called, is presumably limited to certain and specific growth periods which, once passed during maturation, undergo irreversible biochemical events within the cells, changing their pliancy forever. But very recently, physiologists at the State University of New York at Buffalo (Udin and Scherer, 1990) have been able to reinstitute a state of neuronal plasticity by manipulating one of the lesser known neurotransmitter receptors in the brain—the glutamate receptor—using the chemical N-methyl-D-asparate (NMDA) as a tonic for these receptors. In other words, we have the beginnings of a neurological model of a state characterized by an increased ability to adjust and readjust connections among nerve cells, to dissolve and then reset connections, which may ultimately serve as a model of the neurological basis of processes like learning, memory storage and, further, of comprehension and creativity.

What if, we may speculate, we have in the brain, a state-dependent shift, during parts of the sleep cycle, that not only enables the brain to handle its heat and energy concerns, but also allows it a temporary increase in the plasticity of the neuronal connections forming the matrices of memory? Whatever the receptive fields for memory and consciousness are, and whether they are to be conceived of as processes characteristic of the operation of "fields" of central nervous system neurons or whether they are to be looked for in more specific geographic or topographic "sites" within functionally specialized cell colonies of the brain, it is known from studies comparing the function of the left and right cerebral hemispheres, and from studies of the transfer of information between the two, that the arenas of consciousness, memory, learning, and creativity are shaped by both inhibitory influences and stimulating inputs, and that shifts in the level of arousal are further modulating influences of them.

We will be leaving the issue of the role of creativity and sleep at this point, to take it up further when we discuss dreams in Chapter 8. Our purpose here has been to familiarize ourselves with a number of the issues underlying a more comprehensive understanding of the interworkings of sleep and cognition. For now, we will turn our attention to the more chemical side of the sleep–wake cycle.

Chapter 6

It Must've Been Something I Ate
Nutrition and Sleep

For thousands of years in human history various potions and concoctions have been used to induce changes in mental states and to affect mood. In fact, "melancholy" comes from the Greek words *melas* (black) and *khole* (bile). Ancient Greek physicians attributed depression to a state associated with darkened bile. This was part of their theory of "humors," relating body fluids to different mood states. Thus the terms phlegmatic, sanguine, and choleric, in addition to melancholic.

The four basic temperament types conceptualized by Hippocrates and other ancient physicians involved body fluids and their interaction with food. Of interest in more modern times is the Russian physiologist Ivan Pavlov, who revived these ancient categories in characterizing the nervous systems of dogs: the choleric ones got excited too easily; the melancholic ones could be too easily inhibited; the phlegmatic ones were slow to move either in the direction of excitement or inhibition; and the sanguine dogs could move rapidly in either direction without reaching an extreme. Pavlov did not directly link these temperament traits to foodstuffs, but ancient Greek, Roman, Chinese, and Aztec cultures did. In fact, all early cultures developed rituals requiring the use of a pharmacy of herbs and nutrients to modify human behavior, to cure ailments, and to affect psychological functioning. Perhaps Pavlov's apparent disinterest in the "chemical"–nutritional connection reflected his nineteenth century roots and a different model of behavior that had gained great influence, namely the electrical model. It is rather ironic since he won the Nobel prize for his work on the physiology of digestion. And were he alive today, he might wonder at the discovery of the chemical called cholecystokinin, which provokes contraction of the gall bladder, but which is also secreted by neurons in the brain whose chief function is mood regulation.

One might say that Pavlov was trying to reconcile two apparently different views of brain activity by linking terminology from the ancient "soup" theory (humors, fluids, chemicals) to modern "sparks" theory (electrical current). The theory of sparks is dominant among scientists and medical people, while the "soup" theory has many adherents among the various offshoots of folk medicine. That these two formerly diverging theories are rapidly converging, thanks in part to discoveries over the past few years, is a major development in humanity's manner of looking at itself. For, as any student of the history of science can observe, all human knowledge (not just the scientific kind) is built on models which we use to organize and understand our facts, and to represent our current view of reality. The model of the brain as a soupy, damp structure, somewhat like a large gland, that responds to various foods and fluids with which we ply ourselves, served well to organize the prescientific observations of early medical practice. The ascendancy of an alternate, more technological model replete with sparks, bells, and whistles suited the atmosphere following the Industrial Revolution. The first step in understanding the most recent thinking about the relation between nutritional chemistry and mental states such as sleep must begin with a review of the nineteenth century "sparks" model of brain function and the late twentieth century neoclassical "soup" model.

The first upsurge of truly scientific observations regarding the brain as the seat of intellect, mood, and sleep-activity cycles came near the end of the 19th century and coincided with momentous discoveries in the realm of electricity and electromagnetism. When it was discovered that tiny electric currents could stimulate muscle movement and brain function, and when in the 1930s it was noted that the brain itself gave off electric waves, it became fashionable to think in terms of a more or less pure electric model of brain function. Who of us has not seen this model portrayed in one of the many Frankenstein movies in which the humanoid monster is brought to life by a gigantic lightning bolt? At a considerably less lugubrious level, the brain has been compared to a telephone network or an electronic computer. And Sigmund Freud, a neurologist prior to developing the theory of psychoanalysis, called extensively on a more or less electrical model in formulating his theory of psychic drives.

While this model of brain function led to many important discoveries and medical innovations, such as the electroencephalogram or EEG, which can detect epilepsy, tumors, and strokes, it represented only one model of brain function and, therefore, tended to mask the direct role of chemistry in day-to-day functions of the brain. It was popularly presumed that: (1) chemicals, like sleeping pills, tranquilizers, and alcohol, were merely poisons which interfered with the fundamental electrical activity of the brain, and (2) chemical messengers in the bloodstream, called hormones, primarily contributed to gradual, long-term changes in brain functioning and were not relevant to daily variations in brain function. Furthermore, any talk of the role of ordinary foodstuffs or vitamins in the modulation of mood or sleep had been relegated to a lunatic fringe.

In 1973, The American Psychiatric Association issued a justifiably scathing critique on the exalted claims for the use of megavitamins in the treatment of mental or emotional disorders. However, five years later, in 1978, a report in its prestigious journal on the use of vitamin B_6 in the treatment of infantile autism was treated with respect. This apparently dramatic turnaround can be attributed to the development of a new medical model involving the word "neurotransmitter," a concept that has revolutionized the way we look at brain and mind function.

CHEMICALS OF THE BRAIN, NEUROTRANSMITTERS

A neurotransmitter is a chemical entity, a fragment of a protein molecule which serves as a messenger unit from one brain cell to the next. It also serves as the messenger system from our peripheral nervous system to our muscles and organs. A number of molecules have been recognized as neurotransmitters, functioning as chemical messengers both within the nervous system and between the nervous system and other organ systems within the body. One of these, acetylcholine, has been known for a long time to be essential in the activation and regulation of muscle contraction, and many drugs including those in the poison darts of African pygmies have been used to inactivate it to produce paralysis . . . either on the surgeon's operating table or in some jungle battlefield.

Perhaps it is easier to see how drugs operating on the nervous system might be simply conceptualized as poisons. However, things are not so simple. And up until the last few years, it was simply not possible to disentangle the myriad pathways of chemical systems in the brain. Now, with the development of dazzling new investigative techniques, it has become possible to begin ferreting out the secrets of that incredibly compact system. With the help of new fluorescent dyes, it became possible to trace some of the chemically coded pathways through the brain and to record the impact, for instance, of various substances, or even, for that matter, of an individual's single meal on the functioning of these systems.

Today there are several dozen chemical candidates in good standing for the role of neurotransmitter in various sections of the brain, and there is a growing appreciation of their role not only in mood and sleep regulation, but in learning, memory, and intellectual functioning as well. For example, acetylcholine, formerly viewed as active only in muscles, glands, and organs, is now seen to have an important and perhaps vital role in the central nervous system functions regulating the behavioral states of caution, fear, and depression, and associated with memory and learning. Norepinephrine, as well, appears to be involved in myriad functions regulating mood states. The neuroactive agent serotonin is involved in the regulation of impulse control. And the neurotransmitter dopamine, is bound up with the establishment of anxiety thresholds or cognitive organization.

Then a discovery was made that was as startling as this equation between the particular biochemical messenger and the specific psychological state it embraces. Researchers at the Massachusetts Institute of Technology (MIT) demonstrated that the level in the brain of some of the chemical messengers apparently responded directly to a meal containing, in the case of acetylcholine for instance, significant quantities of lecithin, a chemical very popular in health food stores and used as an emulsifier in many prepared foods (Kolata, 1976; Wurtman and Wurtman, 1977).

Before proceeding further, let us take a closer look at this model of the neurotransmitter. First, think of a neuron, or nerve cell, as a tree with many branches, each of which comes into close contact with the trunk or branches of another tree. Where contact is made, there is a tiny gap, called a synapse. An impulse travels along the nerve cell, from the "trunk," out one or several of its "branches" until it reaches a synapse. At this point, a chemical process is initiated . . . for it is across this gap that packets of these special chemical neurotransmitters travel (from branch tip to adjoining branch or trunk) to lock into "receptor sites" on the far side. These receptor sites are analogous to an automobile ignition lock and are activated by the chemical packet ignition "keys," the neurotransmitter. Once the receptor site is activated, the relayed message is further transmitted, as a nerve impulse, down the subsequent nerve trunk.

Thus a chain reaction is mediated by each of these specific chemicals, and the level of functioning of the whole system is, at least in part, dependent on the production and maintenance of these chemical messengers—chemicals with names such as norepinephrine (or noradrenaline), acetylcholine, serotonin, and gamma aminobutyric acid (GABA). It is astounding to realize how marked the "circuit density" in this system is, with the limbs of each neuron intertwined with others, and with a component count exceeding the component count of all the world's computers in existence today. Although, however, it is currently believed that each neuron type is specialized for the production of only one neurotransmitter "key," administered drugs (cocaine, for example) impacting on only a few thousand central cells out of the many billions in the brain, can still affect a broad area of function. These "few" cells are the ones that "broadcast" to all the rest. Such "amplification" mirrors the action of a guerrilla group which, having captured a small radio station, broadcasts panic messages inflaming a far larger population than they might otherwise have expected to reach. Just as there are crucial communication centers in countries, so there are in the brain.

This neuronal "key" story is just unfolding. Already it appears common for many neurons to contain a second "key" related to the first (like the keys of a safety deposit box). This latter key is not a classical neurotransmitter, but perhaps a more complex and specific "peptide" (a peptide being a string of amino acids assembled by the body, according to different blueprints, from some of the 20 different dietary amino acids found in nature). Also within the past two decades, additional "ignition lock" receptors, this time for morphine, were discovered and, quickly thereafter, many locations in the brain were found where the brain's own natural supply of morphine-like substances are produced. These natural "morphines" have been named endorphins, and have been discovered to be composed of strings of simple amino acids, the basic building blocks of all proteins. Thus, each colony of neurons may manufacture its own special brand of messenger unit out of the chemical building blocks presented to it in the bloodstream. And, so far, no natural neurotransmitter has been discovered that couldn't be derived from the raw materials contained in a glass of milk. With a system as intricately interwoven as this, with contending neuronal chemical factories, the brain comes to resemble a grand metropolis, with various messages being sent hither and yon . . . some fast, some slow. Some neurotransmitters (with names like the previously mentioned norepinephrine or serotonin) act in the thousandths of a second, whereas the more hormone-like ones (bradykinin or prostaglandin, for instance) may take hours to days to months to realize their full impact. There is an array of speeds of action ranging, by analogy, from immediate impact, such as that of radio, telephone, and TV, to slower impact, such as that of newspapers and letters, to the ultra-slow such as that of periodicals and books.

Although all these recent discoveries seem to make for a more complex and, in many ways, more mysterious view of the brain and mind, some of them lead to a sudden clarity of understanding. For instance, the ability of acupuncture to induce pain blockade to such an extent that a major organ, like a lung, can be removed while under its influence alone, has mystified the medical community for some time. The traditional Chinese view of meridians in the body seemed like so much mysticism. Then, utilizing the new concept of natural morphines in the brain, it was demonstrated that neurons that carry information about pain impulses in animals could be inhibited by acupuncture, and subsequently that this acupuncture effect on pain-mediating nerve cells could in turn be blocked by a morphine-blocking drug called naloxone. So, these observations then become included in the developing theory which suggests, in part, that prolonged needle stimulation of fine nerve endings in muscle tissue and near joints induces neurons in the spinal cord and brain to produce natural morphines that act as a central nervous system blocker of pain appreciation. Thus, a needle in the hand may, by reflex, induce pain blockade in the jaw through such a central mechanism. Again, we have a chemical transmission system that possibly makes sense of a previously incomprehensible phenomenon and rescues another area of behavioral investigation from the mystics.

While on this point, let us speculate about the phenomenon of "pumping iron" and the "runner's high." Acupuncture studies generally show a delay of onset of analgesic effect on the order of 20 minutes, as if it required this amount of time for those central neurons to get the message and to start pumping out their morphines. Prolonged vigorous exercise as in jogging or weightlifting should lead to a similar if more generalized stimulation of these nerve endings in muscles and joints. After at least 20 minutes of this, many people may well be getting a natural high on their own "narcotics," a high which many report lasts for some time afterwards. The term "jogging junkie" may be more apt than we had suspected, although the cost of such natural narcotics is far below that of the synthetic kind, since it comes down to the mere hundred calories per mile that can be provided by a piece of toast.

THE EFFECT OF CHEMICALS ON THE BRAIN

Even more than some recent illuminations of brain function, is the impact of some rather humbling discoveries. We are beginning to realize that the magnificent edifice of our human brain and mind with its fantastic God-like scope, its multibillion, if not multitrillion part system dwarfing all the computers in the world put together, rests on a small base. Like an inverted pyramid, the cerebral cortex, that vast product of hundreds of millions of years of evolution, rests on the most primitive part of the brain, where cell populations are counted in the thousands rather than billions. As a matter of fact, the brain of the lowly ant has more cells by far than the small colonies in this primordial base of our brain that, although primitive and proportionately small, govern our mood, our activity patterns, and fundamental aspects of our ability to think and feel like human beings. What is even more humbling is to realize the way in which these small populations of neurons can be influenced not just by major life experiences, memories, achievements, and love relations, but also by rather mundane shifts in dietary intake or exercise pattern. We all know, for instance, how drugs like alcohol, LSD, or amphetamines can drastically alter the functioning of the most civilized among us. Yet there seems to be a stubborn insistence by some on ignoring the connection between drugs, chemicals, and foods. Chemicals are chemicals, drugs are chemicals, foods are chemicals, air and water are chemicals. When we look at a beautiful sunset, our eyes begin a chemical process that sends chemically coded messages to parts of our brains where similar memories have been chemically registered and charted. LSD modifies this chemical process inducing distortions of perception and recall, but it now seems possible that very tiny amounts of a similar hallucinogen, dimethyl-tryptamine, may be necessary to the natural process of imagery and imagination. The brain has all the enzyme systems necessary for the production of this chemical agent, and it has been detected in normal people.

Another example: The Chinese have claimed a rate of schizophrenia one-tenth of ours in the western world. Perhaps we can take their figures with a grain of salt, as most epidemiologists do, yet we may speculate that there is more to it. The Chinese staple grain is rice, whereas ours is wheat. The protein in wheat, known as gluten, has a specific amino acid sequence. With what we have learned about small strings of amino acids acting as neurotransmitters, we cannot be sure that certain vulnerable individuals may absorb partially digested wheat protein and thereby provide the means by which the functioning of small colonies of brain cells is distorted. What if these same colonies then ramify to major mood and intellectual centers in the brain? It was 15 years ago when researchers accepted the fact that amino acid chains can be directly absorbed into the bloodstream intact, and that gluten fed to one small subpopulation of schizophrenic patients produced a significant deterioration in their intellectual and emotional functioning—a deterioration that was reversed when the dietary gluten was subsequently withdrawn (Singh and Kay, 1976). A follow-up study suggested that there was notable correspondence between certain sequences of amino acids in the wheat gluten and those found in the newly discovered natural morphines. This finding then led to speculation about the potential beneficial role of narcotic antagonist drugs (such as naloxone) in the treatment of schizophrenia. And so on, and so on goes the logical chain or alternating factual connection and speculative inquiry. With regard to the role of gluten in mental functioning, the jury is by no means in as yet. However, it may turn out that, for some people, a diet rich in wheat may be "overloading" their brains with a neurotransmitter that potentially can distort their mental functioning. The already existing evidence of the "Chinese food syndrome" in some may serve as an analogy: the addition of excess monosodium glutamate has immediate and distressing effects on some people's brains.

If today these discoveries seem self-evident, why has the role of nutrition remained so obscure and cult-bound up to the present? The answer to this, and it is a warning to those who might adopt a simplistic version of nutritionism, lies in the incredible chemical diversity of biological systems to begin with, and certainly of human beings. The reason, for instance, that tissue transplants from one person to another are so difficult is the chemical uniqueness of each of us. With the possible exception of identical twins, we are all chemically unique. Though there are some four billion of us on earth, there are countless trillions of chemical combinations for manufacturing us, that have not yet been tried by nature. What this means is that we do not respond in the same way to the same diet, the same exercise regime, to say nothing of the same life experience. For example, some of us may thrive on wheat and others may become subtly distressed by it. Or, alternatively, many people of Oriental descent have, in effect, a built-in enzyme system which makes excess alcohol intake intolerable, whereas others may have exactly the opposite type of system which actually converts the alcohol in the brain into an opiate-like substance found in poppy seeds. This substance has been found to induce virulent alcoholism in normally teetotalling laboratory rats when fed to them over a brief period. The saying "one man's meat is another man's poison" was never more appropriate than in the light of our present discoveries.

The millions of different combinations of chemical markers on human white blood cells form yet a third example. These tissue antigens, called human leukocyte group A markers (HLA), represent certain receptor sites on the cell walls which are determined by the chemicals which make them up; they are thought to be associated with certain vulnerabilities to diseases such as multiple sclerosis. Here, activation by a common virus, such as that which causes mumps, might lead to this severe degenerative disease of the nervous system in those unfortunate enough to be born with the wrong genetic markers. Investigations today are pursuing the possibility that similar markers exist for all sorts of emotional vulnerabilities.

What this all means is that none of us responds the same way to infection, stress, or diet. Thus, cult diets may happen to be safe for a few people and extremely dangerous for others. Even the revered concept of the balanced diet is in need of some scrutiny. Obviously, those with a strong hereditary tendency toward elevated cholesterol levels in the blood, vulnerable to early death from coronary heart disease, are not served well by the previously considered "classic" American diet of meat, milk, eggs, fruit, and vegetables. This point is rather obvious, and current controversies regarding variations on the theme of what constitutes the "healthiest" diet are beyond the scope of our attention here. But what is relevant to our interest is the recognition that even more subtle conditions affect us all and it is reasonable to speculate on a somewhat individualized diet for all of us as we learn more about our individual nutritional needs. Obviously, there is considerable dietary leeway for most of us human beings as far as mere survival is concerned, but there may be much less leeway when it comes to freedom from minor ailments and mood disorders. It is, of course, this last point that is used by fringe dietary consultants, who analyze hair strands, nail clippings, and other ephemera of the metabolic spoor and conclude with a recommended witch's brew of putative replacement nutrients. These procedures should not be confused with the real and substantive progress being made in the understanding of the role of nutrients in the functioning of various bodily systems.

With all the information and findings identified within the past two decades, what specifically can we say today about the role of nutrition in sleep? Much of what has been discovered about the effects of the "natural" chemicals (including nutrients and neurotransmitters) on the regulation of sleep and waking states has been accomplished by the use of "synthetic" chemicals. Through the investigation of how anesthetics, barbiturates, and other drugs induce changes in small populations of neurons, we have come some way toward understanding the natural chemical mechanism of sleep. By putting people to sleep, we have discovered more about how they naturally fall asleep, just as by building aircraft, we have come to understand more of how birds fly.

To begin with, a French physiologist named Jouvet, discovered a colony of cells in the brainstem which manufactured the neurotransmitter serotonin. He then found that if he destroyed this group of cells, the experimental animal became totally insomniac. However, if he temporarily interfered with this group's ability to manufacture serotonin, he could alternatively induce insomnia, and abolish it by stopping his experimental manipulation. It thus seemed that a sleep substance had been discovered, and from a tiny center in the brain, sprouted a fountain of tracts that extended throughout the entire brain and appeared to be crucial to the regulation of the states of sleep and drowsiness, and even the state of calmness.

THE CHEMICAL MEDIATORS OF SLEEP

When medical science stumbled on a group of drugs called tricyclic antidepressants many years ago, it was discovered that some of these, such as one called amytriptyline (Elavil®), were remarkably effective in reversing the insomnia and agitation of certain types of depressed patients. It was only years later that appreciation began to emerge of the mechanism of their effectiveness. It seems that Elavil® acts to preserve the level of serotonin in those synapses that lead from one neuron to the next in a message chain. In those chains of neurons responsible for the regulation of sleep states, the presence of Elavil® may act like a dam, allowing the build-up of a serotonin reservoir to occur without dissipation, thereby driving the "turbines" of sleep. Much work with other drugs demonstrates that depletion of that serotonin level will produce agitation and sleeplessness, and replenishment will restore calm and a capacity for sleep.

Thus, first, Jouvet demonstrated the role of serotonin antagonists or poisons in producing insomnia in animals; then, much clinical and investigative work established the role of therapeutic drugs in preserving serotonin levels in the brain and restoring sleep to troubled humans. What followed next was some investigation into the natural fluctuation of brain serotonin levels and the relation of these levels to the regulation of sleep, mood, and other functions. It became evident, as a result of these latter studies, that there was a 24-hour fluctuation in serotonin level in the body, regulated by some complex internal clock.

This finding served to further underline an important role for serotonin in the sleep–activity cycle. When serotonin levels in certain areas of the brain are high, as is customarily the case in the late evening, we all tend toward drowsiness. When serotonin levels are low, as in mid-morning, we are potentially at our most alert. Deliberately keeping an experimental subject awake for prolonged periods of time may well induce a reactive increase in his brain serotonin level, as his body, craving the rest and reparation that sleep appears to allow, sends signals to his sleep center, stimulating this increased production of serotonin in an attempt to initiate sleep. After such a period of enforced sleep deprivation, sleep presses most insistently, perhaps because of induced ultra-high levels of serotonin, and he will experience a period of "excessive" sleep—a rebound from his previous state of deprivation. Just as a retail outlet sends orders to its factory when merchandise is depleted, and cancels orders when merchandise is in oversupply, so the state of sleep itself (as merchant) interacts with its serotonin factory in a feedback manner. Both sleep disorders and depression frequently involve irregularities in brain serotonin levels, and, as an example of this feedback effect of sleep on serotonin just mentioned, we note the relatively recent finding that periodic sleep deprivation, of the order of one 24-hour period a week, frequently leads to a dramatic improvement in depressive symptoms in many people.

We now come to the role of nutrients in the regulation of sleep phenomena, with the very recent discovery of dietary methods for modifying brain serotonin levels. As previously mentioned, all neurotransmitters can be derived from the amino acid contents of a glass of milk, and Grandma's advice about a glass of warm milk at bedtime has at least found some scientific vindication. Remember that all protein is composed of varying combinations of some twenty amino acids. One of these, tryptophan by name, is the building block out of which all serotonin is made. Tryptophan is a normal constituent of dietary protein, and milk protein happens to be a fairly rich source of it; therefore, things like yogurt and ice cream are also rich in this amino acid. Researchers at MIT (Kolata, 1976; Wurtman, 1977) demonstrated that a rise in the level of tryptophan in the blood, such as after a tryptophan-rich meal, will, under many circumstances, lead directly and promptly to a rise in both brain tryptophan and serotonin. Here, however, is where it gets a little tricky. And here is where a superficial understanding of this phenomenon has led many latter-day faddists to recommend tryptophan-rich meals, like tuna fish or milk, for the insomniac before bed. It is also here that a blind pursuit of massive doses of presumed "natural" substances, such as packaged L-tryptophan, may also lead to unanticipated problems when the full dimensions of a phenomenon are not really understood.

With regard to the first point, the brain does not simply submit passively to any assault upon it from chemicals in the bloodstream surrounding it. There is a type of toll booth, called the blood–brain barrier, which bars the way for some chemicals and selectively admits others. This way the brain is protected from any sudden onslaught or rapid alteration in levels of substances which might be taken into the body and then absorbed into the bloodstream. Certain amino acids are in competition for entry through this toll booth, and tryptophan is one of them. If a series of amino acids are lined up to get into the brain, and they share the same entry route, they must, in effect, wait their turn. It might be viewed as a "quota" system, wherein a food item rich in tryptophan, but also rich in competing amino acids, may have minimal impact on brain serotonin because the presence of tryptophan is diluted or washed out by the presence of large numbers of its competitors. The chances of any one person getting through a turnstile at a particular time are much greater if they are alone or in the company of several others, compared with their chances when a large crowd is vying with them. So too with tryptophan at the blood–brain barrier. Indeed, many protein-rich diets will lead to a lowering of brain serotonin (with a subsequent alerting effect, even to the point of agitation in a select few), because tryptophan is at a disadvantage for gaining entry into the brain due to all its competing colleagues. This agitation has been reported by dieters on high protein diets.

A further note, and perhaps even more striking, is the fact that Wurtman discovered that a diet high in carbohydrates, totally lacking in tryptophan, will, surprisingly, raise brain tryptophan and serotonin levels. It turns out that tryptophan has a few other tricks up its sleeve, for, uniquely among all twenty amino acids floating in the bloodstream, it is bound, like lint to a sponge, to large protein molecules that are a normal part of blood plasma. Thus, under normal circumstances only about 5 percent of the tryptophan in the blood is freely available to cross the brain's toll booth. Now in a fashion similar to a Rube Goldberg machine, when a heavy carbohydrate meal is eaten, blood sugar rises, a signal is sent to the pancreas, and insulin is secreted, responding to control the too rapid ascent of this blood sugar level. In the process, however, some of that bound tryptophan is freed at a time when no competing amino acids are around to jam up the brain's toll booth. The tryptophan rushes in unimpeded and is promptly converted, with the help of vitamin B_6, and some other enzyme substances, into brain serotonin.

Thus may originate the tropical habit of siesta after a heavy, starchy midday meal. Thus may also derive the increased carbohydrate craving that afflicts some high-protein dieters who may be inadvertently lowering their brain serotonin and inducing a temporary agitated depression. And in certain diseases, such as rheumatoid arthritis, it has been found that there is a higher than usual binding of tryptophan to blood proteins, leading presumably to a chronic lowering of tryptophan entry into the brain, thus possibly explaining one aspect of the high rate of depression in that illness.

Along with the recognition that serotonin is implicated in the regulation not only of sleep patterns, but also of mood and appetite patterns, fluctuations in the levels of the female hormone, estrogen, have been discovered that modify the amount of tryptophan binding in the blood. The frequent female complaint of a voracious appetite for sweets or starches during early pregnancy or several days prior to menstruation may thus be viewed in a new light. This phenomenon may very well stem from a spontaneous, though unconscious, attempt to medicate away the lowered serotonin levels with a big dose of carbohydrate. Unfortunately, the use of carbohydrate as medication tends to carry a heavy fat penalty with it, and it has begun to dawn on some students of human behavior that the frequently observed link between obesity and depression may reflect, in part, this natural reliance on carbohydrate to ease the psychological concomitants (pain and discomfort) of abnormally low brain serotonin levels.

DIET AND SLEEP

Knowing what we do about this dietary connection with sleep and mood disturbances, is there anything we can do to avoid overdosing ourselves with sweets and starches in an attempt to rectify such disturbances? As a matter of fact, it was felt that there was. Over the last decade or so, some clinicians began to experiment with pure tryptophan as a medication, using it to treat sleep disorders, depression, and certain other selected psychological disorders. Some of the studies showed gratifying results. However, there are some problems. There are many different uses for tryptophan in the body besides the manufacture of serotonin, and many different ways in which body enzymes (those chemical units that act on other molecules to break them down into their component parts so that the body may utilize this raw building material) might use and digest it. In some people, addition of the extra tryptophan to their diet may merely stimulate their digestive organs to accelerate enzymatic processes that have the net effect of reducing brain serotonin rather than increasing it. And, as with so many other substances of natural origin, it may have toxic effects in abnormal (that is, large) doses.

This is the problem with the simplistic nutritionist approach, where all "good substances" are presumed to be equally good for everyone. At this point in time, its use has come under increasing scrutiny and is to be approached cautiously. We need only remind ourselves of the relatively sudden appearance, in the spring of 1989, of a surge in reported cases of a rare disorder of the muscles, connective tissue, and blood called the eosinophilia-myalgia syndrome. Unexpectedly, people taking L-tryptophan supplements for the presumptive treatment of insomnia, depression, premenstrual tension syndrome, or even a condition of ringing-in-the-ears, called tinnitus, fell seriously ill with this disorder. Whether the phenomenon was caused by some contaminant in the manufacturing process (the most likely-looking explanation at this point), whether it is a result of the direct effects of tryptophan at high, even toxic, doses (for instance, via metabolic pathways other than those of serotonin), or whether some other as yet undiscovered etiologic agent is operating with this substance, the point is that we must not rush too quickly to easy and fixed answers, no matter how well-justified they may initially seem. New findings must always be subjected to the careful scrutiny of the investigator's eye. For who of the health food faddists would have anticipated such a problem with L-tryptophan? After all, it's "natural"!

To re-emphasize: Our newfound information regarding foodstuff building blocks as sources of chemical messenger manufacture can lead to a new cult of apparently easy answers. Here "self-medication" based on partial understanding of the chemistry involved may lead to useless ritual (or worse). One example: A relatively recently published book has presented lists of foods high in tryptophan, with the explicit suggestion that a diet high in these foods will enhance sleep onset. However, from our review it should now be evident that not only is the situation quite complex, but specifically, a food with high levels of tryptophan but also high levels of other (competing) amino acids, may in fact have just the opposite effect.

A substance involved with serotonin production that appears to have a larger safety factor is pyridoxine, vitamin B_6. This is a truly psychoactive substance that as yet has no discovered toxicity level. Unlike tryptophan, it is not a building block for serotonin, but one of the enzymatic tools that the brain uses to convert tryptophan to serotonin. Many people have reported that they feel calm and even drowsy when taking extra B_6 alone. Since a lot of vitamin B_6 enters our body naturally through food and is also actually manufactured in our intestines by resident bacteria, we do not have a clear notion of average daily requirements of this substance (we have no way of excluding it from the body and thereby determining minimum requirements, unlike other vitamins). For example, there is a well-established, but rare, inherited convulsive disorder of infancy that responds to huge doses of vitamin B_6, yet direct biochemical evidence of a deficiency of B_6 in such infants has not been established. One of the only known side-effects to date of too much B_6 is drowsiness at the wrong time, presumably the result of a too high brain level of serotonin in the morning or afternoon, rather than the evening. Vitamin B_6 taken in the late evening as a sleep aid may, alone, induce a perfectly normal drowsiness, without the need for large doses of starch or ice cream. In any case, medical supervision of any such trial regimen is an absolute necessity for safety.

Obviously, there is no wish to engender a vitamin B_6 cult. In fact, we must constantly remind ourselves of the complexity and variety of different sleep disorders. Furthermore, it should be noted that this vitamin does not always induce drowsiness or calmness, since the brain is far too clever to rely on only one mechanism for any one regulatory function. There are, in our brains, enzymes for the breakdown of serotonin that can act with devilish speed to undo all our attempts to increase serotonin levels. When these are revved up through stress or other mechanisms (psychological distress being one), no reasonable amount of tryptophan or vitamin B_6 can match them, and we must fall back on medications rather than nutrients to control this runaway situation. For just as good general nutrition can, on average, raise one's resistance to pneumonia, nutrition alone is not always a substitute for penicillin.

With all this focus on the neurotransmitter serotonin, it was tempting for some to build an entire nutritional sleep model simply on the ebb and flow of serotonin itself. But for all the complexity of this model, we know that several other neurotransmitters, manufactured in neighboring neuronal colonies, are locked in contention for control of the sleep activity cycle. Like newspapers or radio and TV networks vying for public attention, they compete in a push–pull fashion for the right-of-way and dominance of the brain and mind state. Whimsically, we might label the serotonin colony "The Bureau for Calm and Sleep" whereas another group, "The Bureau for Agitation and Alertness," seems to consist mainly of cells manufacturing the neurotransmitter, noradrenaline (also known as norepinephrine). When this latter colony is stimulated with amphetamines or cocaine, for instance, it can hold the fort of wakefulness for very long periods against the serotonin colony. Sudden noises can activate this group in emergency situations, completely canceling out the delicious drowsiness engendered by the serotonin group. Stimulants like caffeine can lend prolonged support to this noradrenalin bureau as well.

Or chocolate, for that matter. It was only in the spring of 1980 that it became apparent how much amphetamine-like material is present in cocoa and chocolate. Because of this, one may now speculate in a more informed manner about the basis of a chocolate lover's "addiction"! Now, additionally, it is known that other neurotransmitters, such as dopamine, GABA, acetylcholine and adrenalin, may range on the arousal side of the balance, an obvious evolutionary backup system and safety measure, since he who wakes and runs away may live to sleep another day.

Although many stimulant substances have been known for some time, the impact of actual foodstuffs on the alerting side of our brain is not as well worked out as in the case of serotonin. There are, however, two amino acids, called tyrosine and phenylalanine, which are the basic building blocks for noradrenalin, adrenalin and dopamine. These amino acids also show a cycling variation in their blood levels over a 24-hour period, yet discovery of the means for definitely modifying their entry into the brain has not proven to be as straightforward as has that for serotonin. There is no blood protein-bound reservoir of these substances as exists for tryptophan, so that either reducing or increasing their content in the brain is proving to be more of a conundrum. At this point in our knowledge, medications alone seem to be the only means at our disposal for making direct alterations on the functioning of the alerting neuronal colonies. As previously mentioned, however, we can use the presence of large quantities of tyrosine and phenylalanine in most high-protein meals to crowd out the tryptophan, lowering the brain serotonin relative to that of noradrenalin, for instance. This phenomenon is probably the basis for the arousing effect, experienced by some, of a high-protein bacon and egg breakfast. In a similar fashion, a high protein meal in the evening may help to stave off the blandishments of the serotonin colony when the midnight oil must be burned. All this seems to stem from lowered serotonin rather than raised noradrenalin. Such common stimulants as tea, coffee, chocolate, and cigarettes do not increase noradrenalin production, but do seem to facilitate the release of the neurotransmitter already stored in the brain for a temporary lift.

THE "NATURAL" INDUCEMENT OF SLEEP

Now some of the classical methods of inducing sleep in a forced manner seem to have nothing to do with serotonin. High doses of alcohol, barbiturates, and anesthetics produce a sleep-like state, though not a natural one. They do this, in effect, by poisoning the alerting system for a shorter or longer time. It is truly tragic how many lives have been wrecked by pursuit of calm via the noradrenalin poison route rather than the serotonin facilitation route. So far this latter route has been shown to decrease the time taken to achieve a state of light sleep (in the language of the sleep specialist, decreasing the latency times) and suppressing the amount of REM stage sleep, but has not yet been shown to have any effect on the deeper stages of sleep. But thanks to a scientific unwillingness to take things at face value, we have begun to distinguish between the counterfeit (although, at times, necessary) sleep from sleeping pills and the natural sleep that stems from a proper balance between contending neuronal colonies.

However, consider for a moment: why should serotonin be able to persuade the noradrenalin system to simmer down when poisons such as alcohol and barbiturates have such a temporary effect? Perhaps Aesop's fable of the wind and the sun offers a useful model:

> The Wind and the Sun were contending to see who could most easily
> induce the Man to shed his overcoat; the Wind tried first, with force,
> to blow the jacket off; the Man responded by clutching more tightly
> to it; the Sun used gentle persuasion, warming him to the point of
> voluntary shedding of his coat.

Perhaps even at the molecular level there is a difference between force and persuasion!

Aesop's fable would probably appeal to many food faddists who glorify the "natural way" and have made much about food "allergy" and its role in general well-being, as well as in sleep and mood disorders. Unfortunately, they do not distinguish between food "allergy" and food "sensitivity." We know too much now to ignore this distinction. To confuse the two is similar, in medicine, to confusing "infection" with the more general category "inflammation"—confusing a part for the whole, thereby impeding the progression of knowledge by substituting ideology for information. "Allergy" is a specific reaction of the body's immune system, involving the impact of large protein molecules, called antibodies, on alien proteins (be they cells, bacteria, viruses, or other forms of "unwelcome" proteins) and usually resulting in some form of tissue damage. This is but one example of the body's repertoire of "sensitivity" reactions which may include overreactions to simpler chemicals (such as caffeine, alcohol, or sugar) with far less dire consequences.

This distinction is important in evaluating new information regarding nutrition and our health. As an example, this frame of reference is important in helping diagnose the significance of a particular individual's "sensitivity" to an external substance. Additionally, without a systematic and scientific understanding of the basis for certain empirical observations and practices, traditional and folk medicine can degenerate into dogma and irrational cult practices. Many of these cults are seeing a dramatic rebirth in the nutritionist and "New Age" movements of today, where undoubtedly valid concepts are mixed uncritically and insistently with unregenerate mysticism. And, again, fixed mystical formulas and dogma, often associated with a concomitant failure to distinguish between someone who is authoritative and one who is authoritarian, ultimately interfere with the extension of our knowledge.

It is important to remember that complexly interwoven

neurobiological and psychological phenomena such as sleeping and waking are regulated by subtle interactions of the multiple intricate brain systems which mediate between the environments through which we pass daily, and our inner states of physical and psychological function. So, an overly hasty push for some magical elixir, even like that of L-tryptophan with its strong scientifically based rationale, can lead us amiss if pursued slavishly. There can be a high price paid for the premature application, or misapplication, of scientific research.

Finally, the saying "you are what you eat" may have to be amended to read "you are what you eat, depending on when you eat it," if the fledgling science of chronobiology continues to uncover remarkable facts. As previously discussed, chronobiology (from *chronos*, meaning time) involves the study of rhythms and timed events, and focuses on the study of the impact of timing on the biological effects of foods, drugs, and other agents. For example, a recent experiment has documented the fact that test animals died five times as often when exposed to a toxin at one time of the day as opposed to exposure at other times of the day. More positively, mice with leukemia survived twice as long when given a standard drug in the evening as compared with the administration of this same drug, in the same dosage, 12 hours earlier, in the morning. This effect is believed to be due to the influence of previously mentioned circadian rhythms, as they regulate cycles of factors involved in the tolerance to stress, around the clock. It may be that the timing of food intake is a crucial determinant of the substance's behavioral effect—for instance, whether it enhances or opposes sleep. A "stimulant," such as coffee, taken at 6:00 PM may produce rebound drowsiness at 10:00 PM. A presumed "calming" substance, such as tryptophan, taken at 6:00 PM may produce a rebound alertness at 10:00 PM. Although caffeine seems related to insomnia in some people, this correspondence is not linear and the time of the consumption of the coffee may have a prominent effect.

Moreover, taking into account one's expectation of the effects and the dose level, any substance may have opposite behavioral and mood effects, depending on the time in the individual's circadian cycle that it hits the brain. For instance, although as little as one cup of coffee may, in some susceptible individuals, lead to increased irritability and difficulty falling asleep, others may use the warm, soothing beverage as a comforting soporific! In this latter case I would tend to understand the phenomenon, from a psychological point of view, as follows: The warm, comforting beverage is anticipated to be just that . . . warm and comforting; the individual has set the stage with his or her expectations of the effect, and the eventual internal, or somesthetic, cue provided by the beverage with its caffeine load is used by the individual to trigger this stage-setting psychological function. From this, all else follows, and apparently paradoxical relaxation is achieved via a pharmacologic stimulant delivered to an expectant individual who has in many ways already defined the very nature of the experience that is to result. The state of the individual, including fears, ambitions and conflicts, will always dominate his or her response to any food intake over the short run, and will usually modify his or her response to drugs as well. For even a drunk can be sobered by a sudden fright, and it may take twice as much anesthesia to put a very apprehensive patient to sleep for surgery.

In addition to the strength of psychological expectancies and the so-called placebo effect, chronobiology may also be able to explain many of the inconsistencies formerly reported in studies of people's reactions both to food and drugs. It also may be able to provide us with the outline for a reliable guide to the influence of nutrients on the brain. We can certainly speculate that a person undergoing "jet lag" may react differently to a whole array of substances than he or she would under ordinary circumstances. We can also speculate that certain foodstuffs, traditionally reserved for breakfast, were discovered through years of trial and error (leading to folk wisdom) to be most suitable for consumption at that time because of their subtle effects on early morning functioning. Of course, different cultures have developed different menus suited to the chemistry and lifestyles of their respective peoples. We are on the threshold of clarifying many of these interlocking and intriguing questions.

It is no doubt true, to some extent on a molecular level, that we are what we eat. However, it is also true that because we are what we are, and who we are, we choose to eat what and how we eat. Dissatisfaction with medicine's inability to "cure" under certain circumstances has led some to turn to a form of pharmacognosy . . . searching for healing foodstuffs and herbs derived from animals and plants. In our hunger for simple solutions to troubling problems, we tend to jump on available bandwagons that may eschew the painstaking and time-consuming paths demanded by meticulous scientific investigation. For although food can affect behavior (as recognized throughout human history—for example, in *The Song of Solomon* we read: "Stay me with flagons, comfort with apples; for I am sick of love"), the complexities of interactions among different bodily systems are such that multiple factors are involved in the effects of any intake load. Afterall, as a species, we have been around for many eons, and were we to be so easily buffeted about by the vagaries in our intakes from day to day, it is doubtful that we could have survived up to this modern day of diet soda and Twinkies.

A final word. Because it is more in line with traditional ways of thinking, it is easier for us to comprehend food's potential impact on our sleep or alertness level than on our thinking style. We balk at the notion that our problem-solving skills may be influenced by what we eat. Yet, our accumulation of drug experiences should be instructive. We have drugs to calm and arouse, but also drugs that play some role in making some of us worried or confident, trusting or paranoid, elated or depressed. We have drugs to hallucinate by, to alter our time sense, to start dreams with, or to halt dreams in their tracks. We are discovering that we may even have drugs to shift our thinking from the lawyer's analytic, sequential logic to the sculptor's gestalt approach. Does this mean that we can hope to discover a pill or diet to change a slob into a creature of taste, or a sadist into a kind man? By the very fact that the brain deals with multiple levels of information besides chemical ones, we can answer, no. However, a pill or a diet to assist mightily in such transitions is not beyond possibility.

Chapter 7

The World of REM Sleep
One Side of Alice's Looking Glass

Some half billion years ago when the earth spun on its axis somewhat faster than today, days and nights were shorter, and the first metazoans (creatures with more than one cell) were roaming the ancient seas. At that time as well, the moon swung in a considerably closer orbit to the earth, casting a more dramatic light over the darkened seascape. Unfortunately, there were no eyes to behold the sight and thus no witnesses to the awesome oversized nighttime lunar apparition. Yet it now appears that there were indeed blind witnesses whose descendants still dwell in the depths. One of the earth's most ancient sea creatures is the chambered nautilus, a fellow who manufactures a new chamber in his shell as he outgrows the old one. This new chamber has been thought to be a recorder of the moon's changing orbit, for the chamber seems to be manufactured on a lunar month schedule. As the lunar orbit has enlarged over the last 500 million years, the lunar month has lengthened, and so the growing cycle for each chamber in the nautilus has lengthened. By calculating the rate of change of the lunar orbit and by sampling the ancient shells from each epoch, we have perhaps discovered nature's "moon dial," one of the oldest of biological clocks. This is but one of many time intervals that appear synchronized with one another in all life systems on our planet.

We human beings, like the chambered nautilus, are subject to a whole series of timed bodily events, from the obvious 24-hour sleep–activity cycle, to the monthly menstrual cycle in women. Until recently, however, these were the only well-recognized rhythms in humans. The current avalanche of new scientific investigation has uncovered a wealth of new facts and now reveals a complexity of human behavior which incorporates a series of cycles timed by a series of biological clocks operating at various levels in the brain and body, varying in cycle time from 90 minutes or less to 90 days or more, and synchronized like the interlocking rhythms of a grand symphony. Previously, we have been like casual listeners to the musical piece; we did not note all or even most rhythms operating in the music. So too we have overlooked, until recently, that is, a good many biological rhythms present in human beings. We ascribed changes in mood or behavior to personality quirks or to outside events in our experience—in many cases without taking note of underlying cyclic structures in our makeup. It was as if we were to observe the ebb and flow of ocean waves at distances out from the beach and to speculate on their seeming random pattern without noting an underlying coral reef that imposed a special pattern on their cycle. We are now in the process of discovering many such "coral reefs" in the nature of man which, just like the ocean's coral patterns, have been built up over eons of evolution to deal with the special conditions of life on this particular planet.

In one sense, there is nothing new or unique about the concept of the cycle in human endeavors. From the trillion-per-second tremors of the components of basic atoms, to the yearly seasonal cycles on earth, to the multimillion year cycles of rotation of our galaxy, we are dealing with rhythms compounded upon rhythms, compounded upon rhythms. Ancient Ptolemaic astronomy made use of rhythmic cycles in its vain attempt to maintain that the earth was at the center of our solar systems. Ancient systems of astrology are based on an appreciation of cyclic events. Since before Ptolemy, humans have attempted to divine some connection between individual human fate and the changing patterns of the evening sky. Astrology makes much of the exact date of birth of a person, linking his fate to the constellations in the heavens at that moment. Some "revisionist" astrologers have suggested that the date of conception, rather than birth, is the significant one, since it is slightly more plausible that minor variations in magnetic fields, presumably generated by variations in planetary alignment, might influence individual development. Of course, it remains to be demonstrated that there is any measurable biological effect of heavenly bodies, aside from the sun and moon. Hence, the data base on which astrology rests is extremely fragile, to say the least. However, there may be a grain of truth tying month of birth to personality pattern, for the brain has been shown to carefully monitor daily light intake through a special circuit from the eye to the pineal gland (Descartes's seat of the soul). And melatonin, which is produced by that gland during the still of the night, turns out to be a biochemical link between the light and dark cycles of the environment and the regulation of the body's internal responses to these cycles. What with the pineal's suspected role in jet lag, insomnia and mood disorders—namely the secretion of this chemical pacemaker, melatonin, which like at ship's gyroscope, maintains the equilibrium of our various bodily cycles—it is not too far-fetched to speculate that babies born in the summer may go through a different initial entrainment or programming of their bodily cycles from those born by winter light.

This chemical coordinator of circadian pacemaking, melatonin, is normally secreted at night. Interestingly, its production is suppressed by biologically active light (that is, by sunlight or by bright artificial light), and, therefore, biorhythms entrained or keyed to ambient light presumably can be manipulated by changing the individual's exposure to this light, thereby shifting the phase of his internal time-keeping apparatus. For instance, it has been well-documented that many circadian rhythms (like sleep/ wake or temperature) can be "phase-advanced" by early morning bright light exposure, whereas exposure in the evening to such illumination will result in a "phase delay" or shifting of the pacemakers to a later circuit. This raises a whole range of fascinating possibilities regarding questions such as how do organisms determine what time of year it is? We can now speculate that, with regard to mammals, perhaps these creatures note (aside from characteristic temperature changes) the variation in either the span of daylight or the length of nighttime, as these shifting time spans trigger alterations in melatonin secretion in their brains.

In addition, it has become clear that mood states are responsive to changes in circadian cycles. And an appreciation of the biological role of melatonin raised exciting possibilities here too, namely that disorders of mood in human beings may not only be understood from psychological or biochemical perspectives, but may also be seen as the result of a discomposure of chronobiologic cycles. We are currently at the point of detecting such disorders of mood which appear to be sensitive to light and, therefore, we are on the threshold of devising therapeutic interventions for maladies of both mood and sleep using, in the words of Friedrich Von Schiller:

> ". . . tracings of eternal light,
> Upon the hearts of men."
> *Hope, Faith, and Love*, Stanza I

Today, however, biorhythm cults take certain grains of truth and compound them with a magical quest for certainty to produce charts and even electronic calculator devices that will "predict" which days are best in your "cycle" for this or that activity. Despite this danger of the degeneration of curiosity into a search for absolute certainty, a strong tradition of scientific insistence on rigorous proof and constant refinement of information has emerged even stronger than ever nowadays. Thanks to the help of machines that can "sit" and "watch" and "remember," we are able to spot and track cycles that we could only intuitively guess at in the past. And if there is any simple summation of a particular theme of the scientific explosion of the past two decades, it is the appreciation of this concept of the cycle and its role in our very nature.

SLEEP AND CYCLES

Insofar as sleep is concerned, there are at least two types of cycles that have been studied intensively in the recent past. There are the "circadian" rhythms (from the Latin *circa*, meaning around, and *dia*, meaning day) which complete a cycle in the course of 24 hours, and the "ultradian" rhythms in which there are more than one cycle per day. One of these latter ultradian rhythms that has been discovered and carefully described has anchored the most important finding in modern sleep research. The pioneers in the tracking of this rhythm are men named Aserinsky, Kleitman, and Dement. They chose to observe closely, in a laboratory setting, normal people who volunteered to sleep under their watchful eyes. It was through such attentive and meticulous observation that the researchers began to notice a pattern of events, each episode of which lasted for approximately 90 minutes, regularly recurring throughout a night's sleep. They noticed that, in addition to certain changes in the vital functions such as blood pressure and pulse rate, the sleeper's brain wave patterns, as measured by the electroencephalograph (EEG), showed characteristic alterations. Furthermore, each sleeper showed bursts of eye movements of a darting type, both to the left and the right, in spite of the eyelids being closed. Therefore, this phase of sleep was called the "rapid eye movement" phase of sleep, or REM sleep for short. Other names associated with this sleep phase, based on additional characteristics to be discussed, are "the third state," "activated sleep," "light sleep," "paradoxical sleep," and "the D state" or "the dream state."

Let us state more specifically what the nature of REM sleep exactly is, and then try to understand what purpose it might serve. In brief, it is a unique physiological episode occurring cyclically during sleep which is distinct both from deep sleep and wakefulness, yet which shares characteristics of both of these states. It is, for human beings at least, a "waking state" in the sense that eye movements, brain waves, blood pressure and pulse show the hallmarks of an aroused person, yet all the large muscles of the body are paralyzed, so that only a quiver of facial muscles, a twitch of the fingers, and the rapidly moving eyes betray the dramatic events going on inside the person's mind. The resultant picture suggests a disembodied brain, disconnected from the motor system temporarily. In most individuals, the intensity of the eye movements increases throughout the night, as REM periods progress. However, in depressed individuals, the opposite occurs: dense episodes of eye movement activity are more prominent in the initial stages of the sleep cycle. Almost without fail, a person aroused in this phase of sleep (whether depressed or not) will report a dream even if he had previously stoutly maintained that he had never dreamed in his life! Although animals cannot report dreaming, all mammals studied (from ground hog to cat to man) do show the same physiological state and it is reasonable to speculate that visual and sensual images may be activated in their brains as well.

REM VERSUS NREM SLEEP

The characteristics differentiating so-called "deep sleep," or NREM sleep, from REM sleep strongly suggest a "captive waking" state. These differentiating traits can be seen in eye movements (still or slowly rolling in NREM sleep, darting back and forth in REM sleep), breathing patterns (slow and regular in NREM sleep, shallow and rapid in REM sleep), muscle twitches (essentially nonexistent in NREM sleep, and present, especially in the hands and face, in REM sleep), and blood pressure and pulse (stable in NREM sleep, elevated in REM). In addition, the EEG tracing of REM sleep shows a pattern characteristic of the waking state, and, concordant with the picture of an activated internal milieu disengaged from any large muscle groups which might serve as motor effectors, the incidence of duodenal ulcer exacerbations and coronary anginal attacks is increased during REM sleep. Additionally, throughout REM sleep, the EEG reveals episodic bursts of electrical activity that resemble alpine peaks and valleys on the instrument's ink tracing. These are called pontine-geniculate-occipital (PGO) spikes, referring to the areas in the brain where the machine's probes most often detect them . . . these areas are named the pons (from the Latin for "bridge," since it is the connecting span between the spinal cord and the brain), the lateral geniculate body in the midbrain (so-called because of the bulging knee-like appearance) and the occipital cerebral cortex at the rear of the brain. What these bursts of electrical activity, so apparently significant to the REM state, represent, and what the underlying functions that REM sleep may subserve that are reflected by these PGO spikes, is not yet known.

There is a further characteristic of REM sleep, the monitoring of which may, on first blush, appear odd to some: the regularly recurring incidence of penile erections throughout the night, during REM sleep, in all males. But since total or partial erections are reported to occur in 95 percent of all REM periods, monitoring the presence or absence of such a phenomenon gives medical science a new diagnostic tool by which the complaint of impotence may be investigated. Simply put, if a man complains of an inability to have or maintain an erection in a sexual situation, but has documented recurring erections during REM sleep, the physician has begun building a case for a psychological etiology here, rather than an organic one. The investigation of the complex skein of psychophysiological factors involved in impotence becomes increasingly important as our population ages and our reluctance to explore all aspects of human existence decreases, and the qualities of REM sleep provide an additional dimension to this inquiry.

Though the state of REM sleep has been observed in every mammal studied without exception, there are considerable variations in the pattern among species, among individuals, and variations over the life span of the individual. With animals, it would seem that because of the decreased motor responsiveness to external stimuli that is associated with REM sleep, a lot of this stage of sleep might be disadvantageous to a prey species. Always, REM sleep is part of a rhythmic structure in the sleep of the animal or person, but the spacing and duration of the REM episodes can change enormously. About 20 percent of normal adult human sleep is spent in the REM sleep state, whereas 50 percent of infant sleep is spent this way. In the elderly, the REM portion of sleep drops down to close to 10 percent. Some so-called "poor sleepers" show even less REM. The blind show the presence of REM sleep, in varying amounts.

In summary then, a specific, recurring cycle was discovered in our basic makeup. Now, any cycle has a special fascination for us all. Witness the social and religious institutions that build up around cycles . . . from the yogi's emphasis on breathing cycles to dietary practices based on cycles of appetite, from rituals commemorating birth and death cycles to seasonal festivals found in all cultures. Perhaps it is the reassuring quality of a beginning, a middle, and an end with yet another beginning. However, for the scientist, a newly discovered cycle provides an exciting signpost and may serve as a potential vantage point for the closer observation of other phenomena, because where there is one cycle there may be other related ones. In any case, the recognition that a physical state, REM sleep, was linked to an internal "mind" state, dreams, was, first of all, astounding. It also opened the way for the scientific exploration of sleep patterns as they might change over one's life span, of variations in "normal" sleep patterns among different groups of people, and of characteristic changes in sleep rhythms occurring in states of medical and psychological illness—because here was a regularly recurring pattern that could be observed and measured. The discovery of this 90-minute nightly cycle has furthermore led to the search for an equivalent day cycle which some thought might be masked by the different focus of attention and the demands of external stimuli of waking activity. And, in fact, there is mounting evidence for the existence of minor fluctuations in mood, behavior, and even thought processes, again over an approximately 90-minute time span, during the day as well. At the same time, biochemists have been measuring chemical variations in the blood and brain to better understand what happens to us when we sleep. Their findings at first seemed random and shapeless, like a spineless jellyfish. But the discovery of the REM cycle gave them a skeleton on which to assemble their collected data, and the accumulated knowledge began to take some comprehensible shape: 90-minute patterns have begun to emerge in the levels of certain chemicals in the blood plasma, with corresponding shifts in the brain itself.

By now, thousands of sleep volunteers, in laboratories all over the world, have been studied by applying electronic sensors to their heads to detect and record an electric (and, more recently, a magnetic) profile of brain activity during the various stages of sleep. All nerve cells create both a small electrical discharge and a magnetic field as they function. And groups of cells, functioning together, create an electrical discharge which is the summation of their individual activities. The electroencephalograph, with sensors placed around the head of the individual, detects and records the undulating waves reflective of the brain's electrical tremors, developing a profile of the brain's functional currents. This is similar to the function the seismograph performs as it records the earth's mechanical tremors and thereby gives us an indication of the activity underlying the earth's crust.

Probably the most widely used standard for mapping brain activity during sleep, based mainly on these EEG wave forms, divides NREM sleep into four stages or levels of nerve cell activity, with stage 1 being the "lightest" and stage 4 the "deepest." Light and deep are in quotation marks because they are relative terms, but it is a fact that one must pass through "lighter" stages 1, 2, and 3 in order to get to 4. The occurence of REM sleep is associated with stage 1 and usually first occurs after a person has spent some 90 minutes at the beginning of sleep, descending from stage 1 to 4, resting there, and rather abruptly returning to state 1.

Certain minimum amounts of stage 4 sleep seem to be necessary for life, as discussed earlier in the book, and for a long time it was thought that the same was true for REM sleep. However, in the early 1970s, Dr. Charles Fisher reported that one individual, placed on an antidepressant drug called a monoamine oxidase inhibitor (MAO), showed no REM sleep for one year. This person did seem rather bland and banal during this time but showed no other obvious effects. Subsequent sleep deprivation studies, however, selective for REM sleep alone, revealed falling weight despite markedly increased appetite, and an increase in irritability and sexuality in laboratory rats and cats, as well as in human volunteers. The human subjects also displayed an increase in impulsiveness and anxiety and a decrease in ability to concentrate over the 2-week period of their participation. Parenthetically, the fact that REM sleep deprivation might lead to untoward symptoms has led pharmaceutical companies to try to devise sleeping medications that in the course of carrying out their soporific duties in the realm of NREM sleep do not paradoxically reduce REM sleep time.

THE PURPOSE OF REM SLEEP

The phenomenon of "banality" may offer us a clue to a function of REM sleep and its psychological counterpart, dreaming. The reasoning is as follows: as has been previously described, the right half of the brain, in most people, specializes in the processing and storage of nonverbal, pictorial and emotionally charged information, while the left half handles verbal, sequential, and logical material. The right half of the brain has been discovered to be active during REM sleep (fitting nicely with the vivid emotional and pictorial descriptions of dreams during REM sleep, as we shall see in the next chapter). Studies in which one half of the brain has been anesthetized (in patients about to undergo neurosurgery) have shown not only that the two hemispheres process information differently, but that information taken in by one side of the brain is not necessarily shared by the other half when it awakens, again as we have previously discussed. There may be other reasons, apart from anesthesia, for one half of the brain not sharing its experience with the other half. Sigmund Freud frequently noted a "day residue" in reported dreams, suggesting that the remembered dream from REM sleep often contained material overlooked during the day by the left brain. Does REM sleep then represent a "second chance" for the analytic left half of the brain to retrieve previously overlooked information which was registered in the right half? Might REM sleep, further, represent an opportunity for the two halves of the brain to share certain emotional experiences previously masked? Banality in a REM sleep-deprived person may be the consequence of the blocking of this nightly right–left refreshing process, leaving the individual short on color and spontaneity.

Theories regarding the purpose of REM sleep range from speculations about information processing, to the reduction of energy expenditure necessitated by daytime physical activity while maintaining brain tone (by keeping the cerebral motor running at an effective idle), to sentinel functioning in which the sleeping individual periodically raises himself to subthreshold arousal levels to sample the environment . . . like a serpent's tongue "licking" the air. With regard to this last hypothesis, theorists have proposed that, like the scanning radar sweeping the sky and feeding back information about what it "sees," the oscillating eyes of the sleeper, sweeping back and forth behind the filter of the closed eyelids, periodically sample the amount of ambient light bathing the sleeper's environment and report this back to the central control tower in charge of pacing the diurnal clocks. Such a proposition is highly speculative at this point, especially with regard to the effects of varying levels of environmental light on the characteristics of REM sleep, although it has been recently reported that nocturnal animals spend relatively more time in REM sleep than do their diurnally active opposites. But, the fact that light is transmitted to the brain through closed eyelids is familiar to us all. Who of us has not been awakened by the early light of summer? And who of us has not "felt" the shift from "standard" to "daylight savings" time, particularly in our adult years as we find ourselves more sensitive to the changes in ambient conditions surrounding our sleep? If the state of REM sleep provides a special scanning mode to the eye's retina, it is conceivable that this process may provide a mechanism by which world travelers, in anticipation of a time zone shift, may begin to entrain themselves for their new locale even while they sleep, thereby short-circuiting "jet lag"! Finally, concerning eye movements and REM sleep, it is interesting to note that REM sleep seems to be inversely related to the rate of eye blinking . . . at least in the developing human being and in nocturnally active mammals. Specifically, the amount of REM sleep decreases as the infant matures and as the amount of daytime sleep concomitantly decreases; and the rate of spontaneous eye blinking increases from a rate of about two per minute at birth to the adult level which is reached at puberty.

Two evolutionary theories of the origin (and perhaps purpose) of REM sleep in humans arrive at two very different conclusions. One notes that REM sleep is regulated by cells in that primitive part of the brain, the brainstem (part of which is the "pons" to which we referred earlier) which derives from the reptilian brain, and that a characteristic of REM sleep is the "loss" of temperature control. The conclusion here is that REM sleep is a remnant in higher animals of the cold-blooded reptile's state of dormancy which has been carried forward and fused with the presumed newer, restorative, functions incorporated in stage 4 NREM sleep in warm-blooded mammals. In contradistinction to that theory, two researchers by the names of Allison and Von Twyver proposed that REM sleep developed in warm-blooded mammals after the establishment of stage 4 NREM sleep in evolutionary history. They reason this on the basis that REM sleep is absent in the most primitive (and therefore, presumably, more ancient) mammals, like the spiny anteater, *Echidna*, which lay eggs rather than give birth to live young. In support of this theory, some have implied that REM sleep may help to speed the development of the fetal central nervous system in more advanced species.

Let us return to our description of the sleep cycle in humans. During a typical 8-hour sleep session, an adult will have four episodes of REM sleep at roughly 90-minute intervals. The first 90 minutes of sleep is typically the deepest of the night, with a brief

REM sleep stage lasting a few minutes, followed by a descent into deep sleep again. After another 90 minutes, a second bout of REM sleep occurs, longer than the first. The third episode is longer still, and the fourth may last longer than an hour. Most actual dream recall seems to come from this last episode, just before morning waking. Of interest is the fact that REM sleep studies show that dreaming occurs in real time; that is, there is no acceleration in the pace of events in a dream as people once thought. Perhaps this offers a partial explanation as to why right and left halves of the brain cannot always catch up with each other during the waking state—there being so much else to attend to. They must wait for the quiet of sleep to gossip with each other!

To review so far, sleep, although offering a respite from our usual waking levels of activity and reactivity, is not totally impassive. It is periodically interrupted by a series of bodily events, the occurrence of which appears to be biologically determined and which, in many ways, resemble states of active wakefulness according to certain physiological measures. During REM sleep the sleeper's level of reactivity seems to "wake up," but he remains paralyzed and pretty much cut off from obvious sensory contact with the outside world—that is, he remains asleep! He appears to react emotionally to a recreated world that is read out from some internal memory store, as if from some sophisticated video recorder. The internal muscles of the body react—heart, lung, gut and eye—while the outside muscles "sleep on." One might consider it like a giant city which, after dark, gradually shifts its activity so that, to an observer flying overhead, it appears to have wound down for the night. Yet deep inside that city, at many nerve centers, feverish activity begins to prepare for the next day.

Researchers are attempting to detect and excavate those nocturnal centers of activity deep within the brain that may be responsible for the particular characteristics of the REM state. By first studying laboratory animals and then using the data acquired there to look for analogous centers in the human brain, they have discovered a few good candidates for sleep and arousal clocks in the lowest part of the brain, the brainstem. It must be emphasized that, more than most people believe, and more than most scientists outside the field believe, there are striking parallels in the organization of all mammalian brains. Furthermore, at the level of what is presumed to be the most ancient part of the brain, the brainstem, there are equally striking parallels going back along the evolutionary scale to the reptiles, primitive amphibians, and fishes. Although a dinosaur brain has never been directly examined by humans, a comparative neuroanatomist, if given the chance, would no doubt easily recognize many of its features. If there are those who still have doubts about the evolutionary origin of the species, one could simply study the structure of different animal brains, for the architectural similarities are so strikingly obvious that the difference in outside coverings, be they fur, feathers, or scales, pales into insignificance. So it is that we have discovered several centers, especially in the brainstem, crucial to the regulation of sleep and dreaming.

BRAIN CENTERS AND SLEEP

Two centers deep within this part of the brain called the brainstem of all mammals appear to be regulatory agencies and "pacemakers" for arousal, sleep, and REM sleep. Each of these two command centers consists of nerve cells of similar function grouped together as a colony in a specific region of the brain, each is called a "nucleus." The nuclei are alike in that their job is to turn out a special chemical and to distribute it to far-flung regions of the brain. It is characteristic of these neuronal centers that each appears like an entrenched municipal bureaucracy, concerned only with its own self-perpetuation. Each will generate and ship as much of its own chemical messenger as it has the energy to manufacture and raw material to consume. This will continue until, among other things, it encroaches on the "territory" of the other, counterbalancing bureaucracy, whereupon the latter organization will begin what amounts to a counterattack to limit the spread of influence of its "rival." Like the defense and prosecution in some grand criminal trial, each side thinks only of its own needs and may have no intrinsic aim other than its own dominance—but some good is supposed to be met out of this struggle. Each command center in the brain releases, instead of memos, news releases, or other political weapons, a chemical messenger substance that not only influences the brain at large, but serves to hold in check the "excesses" of the competing bureaucracy.

With regard to the regulation of sleep and wakefulness, the first neuronal cluster or command center is called the locus coeruleus (named from the Latin for its deep blue color). Let us call this nucleus the "Bureau for Arousal" because it produces an alerting chemical called noradrenalin. This agent is a close relative of the more familiar body "activator" adrenalin, and is the end-product of a biochemical assembly line which brings with the raw material tyrosine. Tyrosine is a common nutrient amino acid which is part of our daily diet and, therefore, is constantly present in our bloodstream. Noradrenalin is known to function in systems of the brain that regulate levels of arousal and attention.

But were it not for the second command center, the "Bureau for Calm and Sleep," the first center would probably continue to churn our noradrenalin like the broom in "The Sorcerer's Apprentice," causing the poor creature whose brainstem it inhabited to bounce around uncontrollably in a state of constant hyperalertness and irritability (in fact, the affective illness, mania, can be a reasonable facsimile of that very state). However, the system of checks and balances was invented by Mother Nature long before the Founding Fathers thought of it. Here is where the competing command center comes in. The "Bureau for Calm and Sleep," more properly known as the raphe nucleus (from the Greek meaning "seam" because of the linear arrangement of its cells), is no more altruistic than its "competitor," and were it to be unopposed, the brain in which it resided would rival that of Sleeping Beauty. It would continue to churn out its calming potion known as serotonin, to the limits of its energy and supplies. Serotonin is the result of a manufacturing process beginning with another nutrient amino acid, tryptophan.

Happily, each of these chemicals has a sobering effect on the exuberance of its counterpart so that the two systems tend to check and balance each other. These two regulatory agencies have had by far the longest run of any known organization on our planet, having appeared on the scene when the brain was invented some half billion years ago. Their chemical products, noradrenalin and serotonin, are derived in a few short manufacturing steps from amino acids that go back to the dawn of life, some four billion years past. Now, these two brainstem systems are present in all vertebrates ever studied and, through extensive branching systems of nerves, they carry their effects to the farthest reaches of the brain in animals and humans. Thus, though very ancient and comprising less than one percent of all the connections linking one brain cell to the next, these two chemical agencies, intimate neighbors in the brain, one an arousal activator, the other a sleep inducer, play crucial roles in the regulation of dreaming sleep.

Many experiments are now being conducted with various pharmaceuticals, some with animals, some with a previous track record with humans, to ascertain what their effects might be on these two brainstem systems and how these agencies may specifically interact to regulate the sleep–wake cycle. There is still considerable uncertainty in the findings regarding the brain's response to many drugs. Only the surface of the problem has been scratched as yet, but it is interesting to note that several drugs used in the active treatment of psychiatric disorders appear to decrease REM time. Other drugs, such as caffeine and chlordiazepoxide (Librium®), appear not to affect time spent in REM sleep at all, while drugs like the tranquilizer and antihypertensive reserpine and the hallucinogen LSD tend to increase REM sleep. It is becoming increasingly possible for scientists, armed with these pharmacologic tools, to dissect out different functional components of the brain's sleep centers, much like a TV repairman does when, by using electronic probes, he tests alternative circuits by putting a charge in at one end and watching for results at the other.

With the discovery of REM sleep, it quickly became possible to assign certain symptoms of sleep disturbance to a place inside or outside the REM sleep phase. It now appears that teeth grinding, rhythmic head banging and *some* epileptic seizures occur during the REM sleep phase, whereas anxiety attacks, snoring, sleepwalking and sleep-talking, and bedwetting (enuresis) are not associated with REM sleep but occur, instead, during other sleep stages. Furthermore, studies have implied that the physiological state of heightened arousal in REM sleep may be associated with some of the "medical catastrophes" reported to occur during sleep. For instance, certain susceptible people, during the REM sleep phase, may experience increased intensity of the heart pain, known as angina, or increased gastric acid secretion, leading to aggravated coronary or ulcer symptoms. Therefore, a careful sleep history from the patient can be invaluable in developing a more well-rounded treatment approach to the severely ill person. And for any physician who wishes to institute an appropriate treatment plan for any sleep disorder, familiarity with the stages of sleep and with the effects of drugs on these stages is essential.

Today, we appear to be on the threshold of clarifying the biology and chemistry of sleep and wakefulness. Technology is developing at a mind-spinning rate so that undreamed-of techniques for measuring the subtle shifts in brain function, as it relates to environment and its own timetables, are literally within months of actualization. An example is the "CAT" scanner or the so-called "PET" scanner, spin-offs from the X-ray technology. The machine has the present ability to peer into the brain and zero in on any area in order to eavesdrop on the function of groups of living neurons as small as twenty-five in number. Its developers are aiming to improve this precision to the point that the individual cell can be monitored. That this machine alone may increase our knowledge of the brain a thousandfold may prove to be an understatement. The fact that with this thousandfold increase, we will find ourselves with a thousand times as many questions will not be surprising either. Already, refinements of this new scanner are being employed to look for the presumed metabolic derrangements occurring in such scourges as schizophrenia, depression, and learning disabilities. The study of sleep, and REM sleep in particular, will be high on the agenda of behaviors to be evaluated with these new devices. An investigator graduating from the use of the now classical electroencephalograph to the PET scanner would experience something of the mental shock that a stone-age Philippine tribesman might experience taking a ride in a space shuttle.

DREAMS AND REM SLEEP

Despite these mind-boggling advances in research technology, we are still led to ask whether all answers to questions regarding the functions of sleep and dreaming will be found in biology and chemistry. The immediate answer to such a question is that there are different levels at which any phenomenon can be studied. As an example, one can describe a symphony concert from the point of view of the physics of sound and harmonics, the instruments used, the style of music composed, or the personality and presumed intent of the composer.

But it is one thing to describe the subtleties of a Beethoven *composition*; it is another thing to precisely describe one's *love* of Beethoven's music. For, just as all chemical events cannot be reduced to study at the level of physics, all psychological events cannot be reduced to study at the level of physiology and chemistry. From one vantage point in the study of dreaming, for instance, different scientific disciplines (like physiology and chemistry) may supply the words, but where is the music? Having emphatically embraced the concept of multiple levels of knowing an event, we must put our thoughts into action and avoid the frequent pitfall of looking at a phenomenon from only one perspective.

Consider a person who has suddenly been promoted to a new and challenging position in which many difficult decisions need be made, who may then experience a prolonged period of difficulty in falling asleep. On closer inspection, we find that this person has tended to experience promotions as threats of failure in functioning since he was a child, receiving much parental anxiety concerning his school performance, with each successful schoolyear setting him up for the still more dangerous next grade. It would be easy, upon a thorough psychological analysis of his situation, to ascribe his sleeplessness to experiential factors both past and present. If no questions were directed toward other phenomena, the clinician might not pick up a history of sleeplessness with a rhythmically recurring pattern of onset in the fall. The clinician might also overlook a peculiar pattern of seasonal sleepiness in the man's extended family. These latter areas of inquiry are not exclusively at a psychological level but involve a search for possible biological contributions to the particular phenomenon of this man's sleeplessness. The error that can be made here is the acceptance of a plausible explanation, at one level of inquiry, as the whole answer. In the case of the man in question, the psychological perspective may be sufficient for the purpose of clinical treatment, or at least the missed biological rhythm data may not have serious consequences.

On the other hand, if a person has a prolonged reaction to a drug, perhaps based on some biological predisposition but resulting in a psychotic reaction, it may be concluded that he has a personality disorder, that he had an early childhood developmental deviation, and that he will have a very questionable future, if only a psychological model was used for dealing with psychotic behavior. Such conclusions could have a severe impact on that person's future, both socially and psychically. It is necessary for us then to recognize different levels of interpretation of human events and to know that we cannot always assign a single given level of understanding to a given event. Nowhere is this more of a challenge and a conundrum than in the consideration of dreaming, as we shall see in the next chapter.

To return the focus to the physiological state known as REM sleep, we can ask, at this level of physiology, what the purpose of REM sleep might be. Certainly, many find it hard to believe that there is not a difference in function between REM sleep and stage 4 NREM sleep, given the distinct structural differences between them. But how shall one test these functions? Well classically, researchers have attempted to understand the function of a portion of a system by investigating the effect of its removal from the scene. For instance, Dement undertook to eliminate the REM sleep phase from the sleep of volunteers by the simple expedient of waking them up whenever they showed signs of entering this phase. He discovered that, with deprivation, there was a compensatory rebound effect, with increased REM sleep the night following the siege of interrupted sleep. The longer he tried to deprive these sleepers of REM sleep, the more insistent and prolonged was the subsequent rebound effect. These experiments led him to suggest that there must be an accumulation, to some critical level, of some neurochemical substance in the brain during sleep. Prior to Dement's experiments in the United States, the Frenchman Jouvet had manipulated sleep patterns in animals, both by destroying serotonin-producing cells in the brainstem, or simply by temporarily interfering with serotonin production. He speculated that REM sleep might occur at certain points in, and perhaps as the result of, the rhythmic oscillation of serotonin levels during sleep.

Let us now consider the college student who has volunteered

a few nights of his time for a small fee and a chance to further the progress of science as he gets wired up to sleep in the laboratory. Tiny electrode wires record the movement of his eyes and the electrical discharges of his brain as he dozes off. Minutes after he falls asleep, the EEG leads on his scalp record his descent into deep sleep, a phase that should occupy most of the first two hours of the night's sleep. But tonight, something different is going to happen; tonight his sleep is going to be modified (with his prior consent, of course) by a small amount of a common medicinal substance that will reset his "dream clock." An intravenous cathe- ter had been in place prior to his falling asleep. A technician is infusing a small amount of arecholine into his plasma. It is 1978 and he is one of a group participating in a study by Sitaram, Moore, and Gillin (1978), who were able to demonstrate that the onset of REM sleep cycles could be reset forward, like the resetting of a clock, by using tiny infusions of this drug.

Arecholine affects a third major neurotransmitter system in the brain called the cholinergic system (so named because it uses the chemical acetylcholine as its agent or messenger). Inter- estingly, a drug with the opposite effect on the acetylcholine system, called scopalamine (the "truth serum" used by spies in many World War II films and actually found in some cold tablets), blocks the onset of REM sleep for hours. Once the drug inter- ference ceases, however, the REM sleep phase proceeds at the usual intervals and for the usual amount of time. Clearly, the biological clock that paces the appearance of this phase of sleep is open to influence from both the experiential world and the chemical environment. However, definitive knowledge of its final underlying structural nature is not yet within our sight.

REPRISE: THE SIGNIFICANCE OF REM SLEEP

Having addressed the question of what the nature of REM sleep might be, let us turn again to the issue of what purposes this phenomenon may serve. There are many theories as to the func- tion and meaning of dreams (some of which we will review in the next chapter), and following this trend, theories regarding their apparent biological counterpart, REM sleep, have begun to proliferate as data have accumulated. Dement, noting the far greater amount of REM sleep present in early childhood, suggested that the function of REM sleep was to aid somehow in the development and maturation of the brain. An alternative series of explanations proposes that cycling states of activation during sleep are necessary to maintain a critical level of brain function (much like a certain amount of exercise is critically required to maintain muscle tone). This latter family of theories proposes that the major function of REM sleep is to periodically "rev up" the brain during a state of relative inactivity (deep sleep) so that when we do wake up in the morning, we do not do so from a completely cold start.

Still another group of theories focuses on a "vigilance" function for REM sleep. Mammals, as compared to reptiles and other animals lower on the evolutionary scale, have larger brains requiring greater energy usage. Mammals also use large amounts of energy because they are warm-blooded, again in contrast to the lower animal forms which depend on external environmental conditions and need not maintain a constant internal body temperature. In this third theoretical model, sleep is seen as a rest period to permit metabolic repair and energy conservation. Here, it is felt, REM sleep serves as a chance for a sleeping mammal to periodically scan or sample his environment without disrupting the continuity of his sleep. This theory is reminiscent of Freud's psychological proposition that the purpose of dreaming is to preserve sleep by allowing the sleeping animal, man, to handle certain thoughts, feelings, and impulses, occurring during sleep, through the safety valve mechanism of a dream. So, if someone is hungry, he "hallucinates" eating a sumptuous meal in his dream, achieving at least for the moment some substitute gratification. Thus, sleep is preserved.

A number of years ago it was proposed by yet another theoretician in this field, Dr. Frederick Snyder, that REM sleep provides a warming-up state in preparation for a period of brief awakening which might follow each REM sleep phase and which serves as a sentinel. He hypothesized that the degree of danger sensed by the animal during these transitory arousal periods then affects the continuity of sleep; when the perceived threat is great, the preparatory activation present during REM sleep is further mobilized, the organism awakens, and then, presumably, he can more fully respond to the potential danger. It is important to remember that, at least in human beings, such perceived threat may be external *or* the result of internal psychological machinations. This may then form the basis for many sleep disorders in people for whom the adaptive mechanism, originally evolved to allow a sleeping animal to be its own "lookout" during REM sleep segments, is activated instead by some inner fear, solely within the sleeper's thoughts. We have, in other words, evolved to the point of sophistication whereby we respond not only to our external environment but to our internal worlds as well.

At this stage of our knowledge, speculations about the functional significance of REM sleep are just that . . . speculations. Perhaps a listing of some of the factors affecting REM sleep may help to point the way toward where our new-found information is taking us. As we discussed in Chapter 6, dietary intake of the building blocks of neurotransmitters such as tyrosine, tryptophan, and lecithin, affect the ebb and flow of brain levels of these chemical messengers. Such information lends some credence to the folk wisdom that suggested that some vivid dreams were a result of an indiscreet late night snack. However, much more rigorous testing of such hunches will be needed. Clinical studies of sleep in relation to fever and generalized stress are further along the road to verification. Such studies show a decrease in REM sleep under these circumstances. Though the results have been repeatedly confirmed, the implication of these alterations is still uncertain. In surveying the sleep of different species, we can ask why animals of the herbivore type (sheep, for instance) have less REM sleep and the carnivores (like cats) more, while the omnivores (like humans and rodents) have amounts of REM sleep lying somewhere in between.

At this relatively early stage of our knowledge about the active but "disembodied" brain function during the REM state, it often seems that more questions are raised than answered. But such is a hallmark of scientific progress. One exceedingly interesting finding, raising a host of such questions, was that noted previously: the 90-minute sleep cycle seems to carry over into the waking day, with some evidence for a 90-minute mood cycle varying between high-level and low-level alertness. This daytime cycle is associated with variations in blood levels of several chemical messengers including adrenalin and cortisol. Measuring the 90-minute cycles of brain chemicals, whether during the day or the night, is a much more difficult task than taking periodic blood samples, and the technology for such investigations is just beginning to appear on the horizon. When such techniques become available, a whole new host of questions will present themselves for investigation: Does stress lead to an immediate increase or change in REM sleep? What exactly are the chemical shifts in the brain that signal the onset and termination of REM sleep and are there exact counterparts during the waking mood cycle?

What can be said in summary? The REM state is a brain activity organized by a biological clock probably located in a region of the brainstem called the pons. This clock leads to activation of other circuits in special areas of the brain resulting in a picture of partial arousal in animals and the subjective phenomenon of dreaming in humans. Dreams are a form of mental function in humans, dependent for their existence on the underlying biological state. However, REM sleep occurs in animals other than man and we may presume that it serves more functions than dreaming alone, even if animals dream as well.

There are a number of interesting findings that are beginning to take us to the next step, beyond the mere establishment of the fact of biological mechanisms underlying psychological processes. These "second generation" studies with regard to sleep have demonstrated a relationship between information processing, the incorporation and solidification of records of experience (called "memory consolidation"), and different states of brain activation, in this case REM sleep. For instance, it has been shown by a French research team headed by a Dr. Guerrien, as we have previously discussed, that memory acquisition suffers if the individual is deprived of REM sleep, and that subjects experience increased amounts of REM sleep following learning tasks demanding focused attention. It remains to be further understood how different groups of neuronal cells, some excitatory by nature, others inhibitory, respond differentially and yet are integrated into coordinated reaction patterns as the brain shifts among different levels of activation.

The REM sleep–dream interface is an important aspect of the looking-glass nature of the larger brain–mind interface. It would seem foolish for theoreticians and practitioners to become locked into raging intellectual battles among themselves over psychological versus biological bases for human behavior. Both exclusively psychological and exclusively biological theories of explanation are much too current among professionals who ought to appreciate and learn from both sides of the coin. But like the parable of the blind wise men describing the elephant, each camp "sees" only its limited perspective and often chooses to ignore the perspective of the others, to the mutual impoverishment of all.

As we sample many perspectives, from both sides of the looking glass, we can begin to see that various bodies of valid scientific evidence are interlocking modules, interdependent and mutually enhancing. If the history of science teaches us anything, it is that the rigorously examined information, at any level of reality, will, sooner or later, enrich the understanding of other levels. Thus, biology enriches psychology, and chemistry enriches ecology. Great leaps forward in biological understanding of the brain do not diminish psychology let alone human dignity, but enhance it and give it added vigor (just like the hybrid products of the farmer or the plant geneticist). Earlier seminal observations by psychologists and psychoanalysts will prove very useful, in the long run, to the young turks of the neuroscience movement as well (provided they are not too arrogant in turn). This is the intellectual minefield we shall attempt to negotiate as we turn to the phenomenon of dreaming, in the next chapter.

Chapter 8

Sweet Dreams
The Other Side of
the Looking Glass

I dreamt I was being led down a green corridor to a green gas chamber, like Caryl Chessman. I knew the procedure, so I wasn't worried. The executioner was talking to me through a mesh grating, like a microphone or a confessional. He told me to hold my breath when I hear the pellet drop. But, suddenly, I panicked, fearing that maybe I didn't know the process as well as I thought I did, and I didn't want to die!

◆　　◆　　◆

I found myself naked, and I watched, like in a movie, as a translucent self just got up and wrapped my body up in large spinach leaves. I felt more comfortable then, and I became fascinated by a vegetable display of sprouts with little beautiful narcissus flowers growing out of their tops.

◆　　◆　　◆

I was in a car constructed of a rectangle of graph paper, with two people. A woman in a red dress was at a wall, which I thought she was trying to climb. I leaned out of the car and gave her a push. She reached the top and was about to grab a sprinkler nozzle on the ceiling. I told her not to, but she grabbed it anyway. It broke off, and she fell to the ground on the other side.

Glimpses of the future, omens of things to come, repositories of each individual's sense of continuity . . . the meaning and purpose of the dream has been an as yet unanswered source of fascinating speculation, even to this day. From the ancient Assyrians who believed in its demonic influence, through the Hebraic Talmud with its multiple references to the meaningfulness of dream content and the value of dream interpretation, to the conclusion of Rene Descartes in the seventeenth century that "To dream is to think, and to think is to dream," mankind has been alternatingly captivated and terrified by this most peculiar phenomenon which occurs, of all times, while he sleeps! With the advent of more modern levels of psychological exploration and then, ultimately, the ability to identify different types of brain activity and to correlate these with different behavioral states, came the means to make real progress in our understanding of the dream state. And what has been the nature of this progress? Well the pre-Greek Mediterranean world believed that dreams had a life of their own . . . that they existed independent of the individual who dreamt them. The dreamer was but the dream's temporary chalice. Now, 2500 years later, some theorists have brought us full circle. The measure of progress in understanding has been slow, but we have moved from a belief that dreams are external events visited upon, but independent of, the psyche of the dreamer, to a position held by some, that dreams are internal events, generated by the sleeping machinery of the brain tissue, visited upon, yet independent of, the psyche of the dreamer. And this in only 2500 years! But, before more of this, and before examining the dream specimens with which this chapter began, let us first look at the psychology of the dream and dreaming.

The dream psychologists (as opposed to dream physiologists, of whom we shall speak shortly) assume that dreams are meaningful, coherently organized occurrences that make important contributions to the daily psychological functioning of the dreamer. In other words, dreaming represents a form of thinking and will, therefore, reflect different dream contents when different groups of people, with different life experiences, different interest motifs and different thinking patterns (constitutionally determined) are compared with each other . . . be they men or women, children or adults, depressed or elated individuals, African bushmen or Alaskan Eskimos.

Let us return for a moment to "state dependency," a concept developed previously in Chapter 4. With regard to sleep, "state dependent" implies that all those mental processes, subsumed under the umbrella of "cognition" (encompassing systems concerned with language processing, memory, perception, attention, and object recognition), function continuously throughout the entire, varying spectrum of different mental states (from varieties of conscious cerebration to unconscious activity). Only the organizational structure of the cognitive processes shifts as the individual switches from behavioral state to behavioral state. So, just as Aserinsky watched people as they slept and discovered the REM state, Sigmund Freud listened to what people said about their dreams, and from that concluded, in 1900 (p. 506) that ". . . At bottom dreams are nothing other than a particular form of thinking, made possible by the conditions of the state of sleep." As Freud developed his understanding about dreaming and dreams, he constructed a theory that was an attempt to represent no less than a model of the human mind! In many ways, his theory about dreams was the centerpiece of his entire theory of psychoanalysis.

FREUD AND DREAMS

Freud published *The Interpretation of Dreams* in 1901, after his studies in hysteria and self-analysis. In it he established many principles we must understand if we are to grasp the significance of his work and place it within an appropriate historical context as we survey the current status of our knowledge about sleep and dreaming. First of all, and unlike some of the earlier Eastern thought which blurred or totally obliterated the boundary between waking and dreaming life and thereby discounted any cathartic value to dreams, Freud's belief was that dream thoughts represented a process distinct from thinking awake, a process that was important and that represented the operation of a mechanism which attempts to preserve sleep from internal "claims" being made upon it. He developed a theoretical model of dreaming which led to a model of neurosis and neurotic symptoms. He emphasized the importance of early experience (with its wishes, "instincts," and forgotten memories), and he proposed a differentiation between two forms of thinking, called primary process and secondary process thinking. The latter is seen in normal waking, logical, coherent thought. The former is notable for its vividness and fluidity of images, and for its inductive and intuitive qualities with a rather loose and elastic regard for the rules of waking time sense, logic, and causalities. He postulated that the dream is an attempt to resolve internal conflicts between an unconscious forbidden wish pressing to be expressed, and the forces of the psyche rallied to prevent this unpermissible appearance from occurring.

Additionally, he elaborated a series of functions which he called "dream work" and which included functions with names such as displacement, condensation, and representability. The purpose of dream work was assumed to be the translation of the latent content of the dream into the language of primary process thinking, ultimately resulting in the manifest dream, or the dream as consciously remembered and reported. He stated that ". . . the productions of the dream work, which, it must be remembered, are not made with the intention of being understood, present no greater difficulties to their translators than do the ancient hieroglyphic scripts to those who seek to read them" (p. 341). And in purpose, dream thinking was thought to provide, among other things, an opportunity to solve problems, resolve conflicts, buy time, and allay anxiety. Freud thus felt that the dream represented a disguised attempt to fulfill an infantile wish which might erupt while the sleeper's censor-guard was down. If disguised sufficiently well, the reasoning went, the sleeper's mind would overlook the disguised and prohibited infiltrator, no alarm would be sounded, and consequently, sleep would be preserved.

Freud has served as a lightning rod for many modern-day theorists, be they scientific or political. He has been accused of being a psychological misogynist. He has been taken to task for dismissing the "reality" of Victorian child sexual abuse in favor of his theory of infantile sexual fantasy. Some contemporary biological psychiatrists have found Freud's writings to provide them with two particular sources for criticism and "irritation." Firstly, in his essays, Freud often intermingled the words and concepts from psychological observation with those from the natural, biological sciences as if they were completely analogous and interchangeable. Although we recognize nowadays that they are not, for his time they were . . . at least in the sense that they were early attempts to develop some sort of descriptive and metaphorical handle of the phenomena observed. Freud was, indeed, well aware of the limitations of this artifice which was a result of the primitive state of knowledge about the mind and its functions. But perhaps certain present-time researchers, rather than retreating into their own form of rigid parochialism, can learn from Freud's work about the usefulness of borrowing and melding insights, concepts, and perspectives from different disciplines in one's attempt to understand an as yet unexplained event.

Secondly, certain contemporary investigators object to Freud's use of a psychological explanation to describe the "mechanism" driving the dreaming process. With regard to this second objective, that is, to Freud's theory of dreaming, two psychiatrists from the Boston area, Hobson and McCarley (1977), have developed a theory of dreaming based on a biology of the nervous system. They suggest that the normal activity of certain cells deep within the "sleep center" of the brain (located within the brainstem that we have spoken about before) is to spread their electrical excitement to nearby cells, much like one's infectious laughter may arouse sympathetic, harmonic smiles in nearby, unrelated neighbors. The theory continues: Such energizing of adjoining cells results in activity of the systems subserved by these cells, and as a consequence, we see the manifestations of "activation" present in REM sleep-related phenomena. They hypothesize further that part of the function of the cerebral cortex has also been (partially) aroused by the reports from below. It receives inputs from the activity in the brainstem below and, like a factory manager being bombarded by what seems to be an almost random display of bells and whistles on his command board, the brain's cortex then tries to make logical sense out of what is coming in by stringing the inputs together into some sequential scenario. Hence, for Hobson and McCarley comes the derivation of the dream—but a dream with no inherent sense or meaning, a dream without the underlying motivational driving force of the psychoanalyst. Here the dream is but the natural consequence of the half-hobbled, sleeping, upper reaches of the brain, arbitrarily assembling the random inputs with which it is being peppered from deeper within itself. Its job (and here we are referring to the function of the cerebral cortex) is to make "sense" of inputs, and make sense it does. But "sense," in this theory, really refers to "organization." It is as if we had some auditory scanner that might mathematically gather, examine, and then coalesce the subtle blips, wheezes, and hisses of random static into a patterned display on the oscilloscope screen . . . not because there was any inherent "sense" in the static, but because this is what the scanner does—it makes patterns from snippets of inputs!

It most certainly is true that the underlying stuff of dreams may come from random neuronal discharges mandated by forces no more motivationally driven than are those of electrolyte shifts across neuronal membranes leading to "spontaneous" neurological discharges. Putting aside the issue of what the mechanisms might be that determine the timing and occasion of these discharges, we still can find meaning within the dream process. This can be found in the particular sort of cognitive activity, occurring while we are awake, but also during the cyclical episodes of sleep, that is, characteristic of all human higher cortical functioning—namely, the inherent tendency to make sense out of inputs. The dream may not arise, as Freud had initially suggested, in response to a "push from below," as an attempt to prevent the eruption of psychological processes which might disrupt sleep. But curiously, although absolutely objecting to this formulation of Freud's, Hobson and McCarley seem to have inadvertently swallowed his argument hook and line, if not sinker . . . if the manifestation of one's entire argument being significantly colored by the opponent's position is any indication: "Meaning," in fact, can be "imposed from above." You or I take a conglomeration of disparate facts (or "inputs") and impose a system, a meaning on them which results in an amalgam incorporating the stimuli and our own idiosyncratic sense of order (which is derived from, and reflective of, our pasts, our selves). To hold that dreams are without meaning seems simplistic at best and an overreaction in favor of the new biology of neuroscience. Yes, **dreaming** occurs within the brain and is triggered and regulated by impersonal biological and biochemical mechanisms which we are just beginning to understand. But **dreams**, the products of these processes, are phenomena with broader implications for other realms of inquiry and function.

For example, what of the commonly observed case that dreams of men and dreams of women, although exhibiting much overlap, can differ characteristically both in style and in content?

Fingerprints are not the only biological billboards advertising our individual distinctiveness. Styles of thinking characteristically distinguish individuals from each other and, if you combine this with the uniqueness of individual experience and the variability that must be inherent in the different memory systems of different individuals, you can hardly dismiss the importance, let alone the reality, of "meaning" in human life, regardless of how intricate or obscure the blueprint for understanding it appears. Let us not, in our enthusiasm for modern technological advances that provide us with the opportunity to get a biological handle on elusive psychological and mental phenomena, throw out the baby with the bathwater. Let us avoid a descent into revisionist dogmatism which can be nonproductive and stultifying, whether it derives from a rabidly positivistic antimystical position or a narrow and blinded holistic, "new age" stance. True understanding of complex phenomena of human existence, like the consequences of cognitive brain activity on behavior in the case of dreaming and dreams, lies in first understanding the events and then assembling a pastiche from many different perspectives to achieve a coherent picture incorporating both biological and psychological theory.

Whether the internal biologically determined dreaming "generator" of Hobson and McCarley, the past psychological history of the individual, or individual elements of temperament and cognitive style determines the primacy of a particular dream's format and occurrence, we must avoid degenerating into a chicken–egg type of argument. Whether or not internally created signal information provides the matrix upon which the cyclically driven dream state sculpts a dream, dreams have meaning—both within a biological context and within a psychological one. Whether we start from the "psyche" or the "brain," from the "mind" or the "body," neither can be reduced to the other. Both provide relevant perspectives for understanding the nature of sleep.

THE FUNCTION OF DREAMS

Theories about the purpose and function, not to mention the very nature, of dreaming abound in profusion nowadays exceeded only by the panoply of theories generated to account for the purpose of sleep itself. They range from (1) theories likening the dream state to a situation in which the brain finally has some time to itself, to do housekeeping and sorting and filing away traces of those events which are to be invited into memory's permanent gallery, to (2) state-dependent theories which hold that the brain temporarily regresses to a more primitive developmental state during sleep, allowing the emergence of processes which were indeed more prominent when the individual was less cognitively mature, to (3) theories that regard the sleep state as permitting differential access to the right cerebral cortical hemisphere (compared with the dominance of left hemispheric functioning during the waking state). With regard to varieties of this last proposal, sleep is assumed to allow particular access to memories stored in the right hemisphere which, by their very nature, are notable for their visual vividness, primitive thinking style (with a predominance of imagery over logic, and a disruption of a waking sense of temporal sequence and continuity) wherein meanings become multiple and condensed into themselves, and multiple ambiguous meanings and emotional states can coexist. In this context, it is assumed by some theorists that a functional disengagement of right and left hemispheric function occurs during REM sleep and it is this uncoupling which is then hypothesized to be the permissive mechanism which allows events of the day to be integrated with memories of the past and thereby result in a new amalgam of information and possible strategies. It is here, in this theorizing, that thoughts of left–right brain function, learning, creativity, sleep, and dreams all come together.

There are other theories as well . . . most, variations on the theme that nature has developed a means for processing and formulating information during sleep which requires heightened brain activity but not conscious wakefulness . . . that is, REM sleep. Of course, it remains to be seen whether the specific energy requirements for such processing really are met in the REM state or, for that matter, exist at all. Winson, in 1985, wrote extensively about this and, earlier, Crick and Mitchison proposed a plumber's-eye view of the purpose of REM sleep and dreams: to clean out the cerebral "pipes," flushing them of irrelevant, haphazard and nonconstructive cortical connections made during the rush of the previous day's conscious and waking activity.

A bit of neurophysiological information to add to this picture: Just below half of the cerebral cortex on either side lie two neurological structures which in profile resemble the outline of a seahorse. Each is called a hippocampus. They are involved in information processing functions, such as learning and memory. How do we know? Because during learning tasks, one can record an increase in a particular form of electrical activity, with a specific wave-like signature on the EEG tracing taken over the hippocampus. This activity has been labeled "theta rhythm" and is distinguished from other characteristic wave forms like "alpha waves," "beta waves," and "PGO spikes." Now, in addition, theta rhythm can be recorded from the hippocampus during REM sleep, thereby implying that this information-processing "marker" reveals such activity going on outside of the waking state.

Both Winson and Crick and Mitchison have questioned whether two different brain structures oversee information processing during different behavioral states . . . the hippocampus during sleep and the frontal cortex during waking hours. The function of the anterior part of the cerebral cortex, the so-called frontal lobes (left and right) has been established to be that of organizing and overall monitoring of cognitive activities. If there were to be a specific seat for the conscience, that black-robed psychic judge, it would no doubt be in the frontal lobes where this "superego" can oversee and modulate information from both within and without, from the internal environment and the external world, maintaining connections among the underlying emotional and arousal systems of the brain and the motor/verbal/logical and sensory/imagistic/spatial functions of the left and right cerebral hemispheres. It is important to remember here, as we cover the range of theoretical speculations regarding the interplay between neurophysiology and the phenomenon of dreaming, that there may be quite a significant difference between what stimulates a dream to be initiated, what factors then determine how the tale is spun out, and what mechanisms are called into play to enhance the elaboration, recall, and recounting of the dream. An entire series of processes are called into play, only one of which may involve the differential functioning of the cerebral hemispheres, or the cyclical firing of sleep pacemaker cells deep within the brainstem below.

NIGHTMARES

In no place more than in the realm of dream disturbances can we see so clearly the necessity to play in both arenas, the biological and the psychological. For here we must explain not only phenomena such as night terrors and dream anxiety attacks (the latter—better known as nightmares), we must also be prepared to answer why the very themes and mental contents of one particular night's dreams tend to remain rather consistent, compared with the thematic constituents of dreams over different nights. Certainly it is known, both from data gathered in the experimental laboratory and from data culled from anecdotes of daily living, that experiences prior to sleep can affect dreams. It is possible, for instance, to change dream content by hypnotic suggestion (even for that matter, by presleep suggestion alone, done properly and in the right individual), and by presleep exposure to a stressful event which is personally relevant to the individual . . . otherwise, of course, it might not be really experienced as "stressful." If adaptation to a particularly stressful event does not occur before the individual falls asleep, it has been shown that aspects of this event become incorporated into dreams, suggesting to some investigators that they are witnessing the attempt to master the trauma through a mental reworking of selected remnants of the event. In fact, it has been suggested by two Canadian sleep researchers, Wright and Koulack (1987), that following dreams over time, and noting when the thematic content shifts, may give an indication as to when mastery over a traumatic event has occurred. There seems to be no question about the physiological interaction possible between waking states and REM sleep. Although the specific mechanisms by which material from daily waking experience influences dream content are not known, there is no question that such matter can be incorporated into the dream products of REM sleep.

And the question is important for the clinician confronted by a patient suffering from repetitive frightening dreams associated with an agonizingly intense sense of realness: Should the patient be referred for psychotherapeutic exploration of the psychological underpinnings of this symptom? Is there a question of a post-traumatic stress syndrome? Should the individual be referred to a sleep laboratory to rule out disorders such as nocturnal epilepsy, central sleep apnea, sleep paralysis, or hypnopompic hallucinations (which we will discuss later in this chapter and in Chapter 9)? Should drugs be instituted in an attempt to suppress the troublesome REM state?

Repetitive nightmares have been attributed to the artistic temperament, to the chronically psychologically disturbed or to the demon-possessed. Derived from the Anglo–Saxon word for "demon," the nightmare is distinguished from the night terror in that the vivid details remain even after awakening. The night terror (or *pavor nocturnus*) is most often a phenomenon of childhood which occurs during NREM sleep, generally within the first third of a night's sleep, and generally limited to one attack per night. The attack usually starts with a sudden, bloodcurdling, panicked scream and signs of intense agitation, muscle tension, marked confusion, and disorientation. The child may sit up or get out of bed but, for the 30–120-second duration of the episode, remain unresponsive to any attempts at outside intervention. Following the attack, there is usually at least a partial amnesia for the episode. It is thought that lags in central nervous system development may predispose certain children to an instability of the arousal mechanism such that, in the presence of emotional conflict and/or fatigue, these individuals can surge suddenly up from the depths of stage 4 NREM sleep in one of these intense disoriented fear attacks. Although there is a history of these episodes running in families, they are outgrown usually rather quickly. And for those rare occasions where the episodes occur three or more times per week, temporary pharmacologic intervention with the tranquilizer diazepam can be quite successful.

Nightmares are another story. Although also providing signs and symptoms of activation like night terrors, these events occur during REM sleep, not during NREM sleep; and they are almost always associated with vivid and intense recollections of the dream's details, not with amnesia. In fact, 50 percent of people having nightmares not only remember their dreams but report recurrent themes in them. Their occurrence is not limited to any particular age range, and they do not manifest the same degree of panic symptoms as do night terrors. They are common in childhood, and change in character and content as a child moves through different developmental cognitive stages, making increasingly more distinct differentiations between inner fantasy and external reality.

There are a small number of adults who suffer from chronic nightmares. They are thought to have difficulty dealing with hostility and resentment, and, as a group, to be characterizable as distrustful, alienated, and overly sensitive to the reactions of others. Whether this observation can be considered "cause" (that is, following the influence of personality factors on dreaming phenomena), or "effect" (the consequence of living with recurrent bad dreams), or some combination of both, remains to be determined. An additional occasion in which we might see an undue presence of nightmares is after the experience of a particularly distressing event, like a life-threatening experience or a traumatic occurrence which goes beyond the pale of usual daily existence. Such reactions in the past have been called war neurosis or shell shock and today are collected under the title of "post-traumatic stress syndrome". . . a generalized aroused state noted for the presence, in addition to recurrent nightmares, of emotional jumpiness, irritability and inconstancy, depression, sleep disturbances, memory flashbacks to the traumatic event and fugue-like states of mental dissociation and detachment.

The typical nightmare lasts as long as the typical dream, only its content is more marked by the presence of bad feelings— frustrating physical activity, unhappiness, fear, and, curiously, vivid colors. Various sleep researchers (including Jouvet, Hauri, and Dement, among others) have, over the years, described different categories of nightmares, the most frequent of which have themes related to falling, being attacked, or witnessing the threat to or attack of a loved one. Speculations regarding the "meaning" of such themes have been suggested by many. Books abound with overly simplistic psychodynamic menus and interpretation guides to one's dream life . . . fear of falling being equated with fear of loss of love and associated with a history of being unable to show defiance to one's parents and difficulties separating them; or fear of attack being equated with a fear of criticism and of bodily harm and associated with difficulties in making intimate attachments to others, and so on. But beware! We are not such simple creatures that we can all be boiled down to a handful of pat formulas which will then provide meaningful insight into the individual richness of our separate realities. Again, in the pursuit of giving meaning to the experiences of our lives, let us not fall prey to the siren call of popularized and half-baked claims of certainty, be they in the form of archetypal images or of fast-order prescription.

THE MEANING OF DREAMS

Knowledge and self-knowledge are hard to come by. They take time and respectful attention. Dreams are a potential source of such information, but not by mysterious ritual. The other side of the coin does not hold either: It is not sufficient for the parochial biological psychiatrist to rail against an admittedly dated metaphor established by early psychoanalysts in a Victorian era as they struggled to understand how the conscious interpretation of brain activity was translated into a particular individual's particular dream. In fact, Sigmund Freud was the first who had the courage to ask in a scientific way about the meaning of dreams. Freud's adherence to scientific principles has been too little recognized in many circles. His was not the science of the laboratory or the "double blind study," but the naturalist setting more familiar to the ethologist or the anthropologist. His credo, that one learns about dreams from the dreamer, is in the highest scientific tradition, and would be wisely adhered to by subsequent students of the dream. Within this context, we can see from his writings how Freud began to understand the dream:

> The dream-thoughts and the dream-content are presented to us like two versions of the same subject matter in two different languages. Or, more properly, the dream content seems like a transcript of the dream-thoughts into another mode of expression, whose characters and syntactic laws it is our business to discover by comparing the original and the translation. The dream-thoughts are immediately comprehensible, as soon as we have learnt them. The dream-content, on the other hand, is expressed as it were in a pictographic script, the characters of which have to be transposed individually into the language of the dream-thoughts. If we attempted to read these characters according to their pictorial value instead of according to their symbolic relation, we should clearly be led into error. Suppose I have a picture-puzzle, a rebus, in front of me. It depicts a house with a boat on its roof, a single letter of the alphabet, . . . we can only form a proper judgement of the rebus if we . . . try to replace each separate element by a syllable or word that can be represented by that element

> in some way or other . . . A dream is a picture puzzle of this and our predecessors in the field of dream-interpretation have made the mistake of treating the rebus as a pictorial composition: and as such it has seemed to them nonsensical and worthless.
>
>   Sigmund Freud, *The Interpretation of Dreams*

Although his approach here is "psychological," and he went on to propose that dreams were the manifestations of unconscious wishes which had been reworked and disguised by a hypothesized "censor," Freud was a neurologist and no stranger to the brain. As such he would be delighted with the newer findings on the physiological side of the looking glass. But it is, again, important to emphasize that the observations about the way people think can supply us with important data regarding the structure of the brain, and reported dreams are at least as important sources of data as are the squiggles of lines on an electroencephalograph. Freud passionately believed that dream analysis provided the "royal road" of access to understanding the functioning of the unconscious mind. His two major discoveries in this regard were (1) that dreams are understandable according to a principle he called psychological determinism—that is, what we think about, muse about, and dream about is influenced in a direct way by prior stimuli, inputs, and experience, and (2) that the characteristics of thought in sleep, revealed through dreams, are different from those during waking hours: linear time dissolved, pictorial representation gained ascendancy over more auditory, word-based thinking, one image seemed to represent many different meanings, all of which were relevant to the dreamer but were telescoped into the one reflection. These different meanings are inapparent at first until, like the still bottle of club soda sitting on the shelf which reveals nothing of the contents compressed within it until uncapped, the dreamer begins to freely associate with the dream image and thereby draws thought connections between it, his previous life events and the feelings they evoke, and his reservoir of stored memories.

The useful fact about dreams, namely that they occur during sleep when, presumably, conscious censoring of thoughts is at low tide, gives us a window through which to peer at the content of an individual's psychological universe, if only we follow the key. And the key is really a painstaking process involving, at its core, the use and analysis of freely associated material. From the clues and hints of the "rebus puzzle," we reconstruct the message. Of course, as you can see, we can perfectly well pursue understanding at this level of psychological inquiry even as we simultaneously pursue inquiry at the neurobiological level regarding the triggers and modulators of the sleeping cycle itself. And although it is generally acknowledged that Freud's teleological hypothesis (that the function of dreaming is to preserve sleep by incorporating, and thereby neutralizing, disruptive stimuli, whether they be from within or from without) was more of a romantic notion based on the limited appreciation, in Victorian times, of the neurophysiology underlying REM sleep, it has to be recognized that dream thoughts do maintain some significant continuance with waking thinking, even if the connection is concealed at times. Also, although the very purpose of dreaming may not be to preserve sleep, even as an adjunctive psychological manifestation of the organismic REM state, it may still serve an adaptive function, a portion of which may happen to be the preservation of sleep!

Modern-day critics of Freud's dream theory hypothesize a biological function for dreams, not a psychological one. For contemporary critics like Hobson and McCarley (1977), meaning in dreams is only constructed after the fact by a cerebral cortex trying to make sense out of images generated from the biological cauldrons below. However, modern-day psychoanalysts for their part emphasize the subtle and creative endeavors of the dreaming brain and further maintain that such activity continues into waking life as the dream is further reworked in the process of relating it to another person. In fact, there are researchers who suggest more than a romantic link between dreams and certain forms of creative achievement. The classic example of Kekule and his discovery, through a dream, of the chemical structure of the benzene ring, is probably just the tip of the iceberg. It may turn out that many forms of visual creativity are in some way connected to the process of dreaming.

Whether the inner, biologically determined dreaming "generator," the historical repository of past psychological experience, or the determinants of an individual's perceptual and cognitive style decide what form a dream will take and when it will occur, we had again best avoid the chicken-and-egg type of argument. Whether the centers deep within the brainstem create a biological matrix upon which a dream's psychological elements are hung, or whether the dreamer's psychological history and experience provide the armature upon which the cyclically driven D-state sculpts a dream, dreams have meaning, both within a biological context **and** within a psychological one. Again, whether we start from the "psyche" or the "brain," the "mind" or the "body," neither can be reduced to the other. Both provide relevant perspectives for understanding the nature of sleep and dreams. For those who would try to reduce mental states to mere organ events, further explication is lost rather than gained by this jumbling of observations from two different levels of inquiry, and by the mixing up of terms from both. One can then rapidly fall into the trap of using the language and observations derived from one level to explain the consequences in another level. This has been pointed out by others, and a fanciful variation on this theme was used by the author Stephen King in his novel *The Talisman*, a fantasy/adventure story in which the protagonist is caught shuffling between two realms of reality.

DREAMS AND RECALL

When we begin to consider both the biological and the psychological substrates for the dreaming phenomenon, we inevitably are brought to the issue of remembering, or for that matter, forgetting dreams. With the advent of techniques for monitoring the phases of sleep and the consequent recognition of REM sleep and its attendant state of brain arousal, it became apparent that the mentation that accompanies dreaming must, too, be a regular concomitant of the REM state and, therefore, that we must dream more than we remember. Of course then, one wonders how pervasive forgetting of dreams must be among individuals, although processes other than motivation of temperament could be at work accounting for such differences . . . like insufficient stimulus from the dream or insufficient relevance of the dream to command a focus of attention and cross an awareness threshold, or time delays and memory decays, or other as yet unidentified metabolic or neuroregulatory events occurring during sleep phases and varying from day to day.

But from early on, and certainly from the early writings of Freud, the behavioral scientists' primary assumption was that dreams are forgotten and, from a psychoanalytic point of view, this forgetting was assumed to be purposeful, compelled by a psychological force called "repression." It was as if a censoring "Puck-like" character, perched at his intracerebral judicial bench, viewed the proceedings of the dream production, found their contents unacceptable for conscious awareness, and either "bleeped" them out or masked them, thereby preventing conscious retrieval from short-term memory stores. Not only was the dream thereby "x-rated," it was removed from the store's shelves and placed in a deeper, more inaccessible repository.

Nowadays, we know more about how the interrelated phenomena of learning, remembering, and forgetting handle subject matter which is controversial for the individual. We know that factors which affect memory while awake have similar effects on dream recall. In addition, there are indications that some individuals may be distinguished from others by the presence of a constellation of traits collectively called "field dependence" (or its counterpart, "field independence"). This category refers to a perceptual style in which one is able to detect, on psychological testing, a simple figure embedded within a complex figure; or, when taken into other arenas of psychological perception, it refers to the ability to use one's own gravitational sense of orientation in the presence of confounding external environmental cues (like the small aircraft pilot or the scuba diver disoriented by various visual, auditory and tactile cues in an "alien" environment but maintaining a field-independent sense of "which end is up"); or, in an interpersonal sense, the ability to differentiate one's self from the imposed external pressures resulting from the expectations of others. In other words, the field-dependent individual cannot see the trees for the forest. And it has been thought by some that the characteristic of field dependence/independence may differentiate poor dream recallers from good ones. If so, then the key underlying factor may not be the complex construct of memory regulation, known as repression, but much more simply a greater susceptibility to distraction, particularly during shifts from one mental state to another.

Investigations so far suggest that distractions, a delay in

reporting a dream coupled with limited salience of the dream subject matter and meager emotional content, and a less aroused mood prevailing before sleep can all interfere with dream recall. With regard to this last point, it is interesting to note that "arousal" can come in many guises, not the least of which is presleep upset. Since we presume a continuity of mental activities (perhaps changing in quality as shifts among different mental states occur), we would have to assume that the turmoil and coping mechanisms set into motion just prior to sleep do not just stop dead in their tracks just because we go to sleep . . . even though that may be the desired outcome! Therefore, turmoil before sleep may be quite "activating," neurologically speaking, perhaps increasing one's inward attention and dream activity. We might speculate that herein lie the seeds from which might spring the fruitful idea that sleep and dreams lead to creative problem-solving.

So, while dream researchers are pursuing the answers to the puzzle of dream recall, you can begin your own subjective, introspective study. Notice which dreams you do recall. What are the circumstances immediately surrounding the times that you awaken from a dream you recall? Are you the kind of person who is easily distracted in general? Was the awakening time in question devoid of such distractions? Was there a particular importance or notability to you regarding the content or feeling of the dream?

Incidentally, a further note about the physiological mechanisms which may contribute to the ability to recall dreams. Much of purposeful, conscious recall is thought to be seated primarily in the left cerebral hemisphere and a number of researchers have pointed out the difference among individuals regarding their images and illustrations of a dream's story, on the one hand, and the very story line, or narrative, of the dream on the other. So, different functions for the left and right cerebral hemispheres have been suggested, not only in the storage of memories and style of thought processing (which we discussed in previous chapters), but also with regard to the handling of the dream . . . that is, the recall, elaboration, and reporting of the dream.

Probably both psychological and physiological factors determine the degree of dream recall and the attempt, again, is to identify processes within which these factors may be played out. Not everybody can put impulses into images with equal facility, or felicitously, then turn these images into words. These procedures, like other intrapsychic processes, are subject to individual variability. It has been assumed that the same general forces involved in memory in waking life are responsible for the recall of dreams. To what extent this is so is not yet known. Certainly part of the recalling process involves the ability to verbalize or "name" an impulse or experience that has not yet achieved the status of full attentive consciousness. Although the interplay between the experience of consciousness and the neurophysiological focusing or attention mechanisms involved in this experience is complex (and mutually interactive so that which is cause and which is effect cannot be readily determined), and although the process of dreaming may take place independent of the things dreamed about, neither recognition justifies the conclusion that dreams themselves are random in content, nor that how they are handled by the dreamer is a random process.

A lot of research and speculative fingers are beginning to point to the forebrain as the neurophysiological seat of many of the processes involved in the experience of "consciousness" and in mechanisms of recall as well as the selective screening process called forgetting. This anterior cerebral cortex, which appears to be the final arbiter of much that we experience as "conscious" and much that we experience as logic- and syntax-bound, may be influenced, in a state-dependent fashion, by the operation of other brain centers and other brain states. As an example, if one is asleep with right hemispheric processes in ascendancy, the forebrain's conclusions (based on its own *Robert's Rules of Order*) will be different from those present if the left hemisphere's more logical world view is functioning. An alternative theoretical perspective can be seen in Laurence Miller's (1989) essay "On The Neuropsychology of Dreams," in which he suggests that what distinguishes "night dreams" from "day dreams" is the preservation of frontal lobe function in the latter and the suspension of such function in the former. In either case, daydreams may provide clues to underlying desires, puzzles, and fears, as well as an additional dimension for the imagination to operate (if such a process may be attributable to the frontal lobes) . . . not just an escape from daily drudgery or boredom. And transitional states of frontal lobe function, during the light stages just at the beginning of descent into sleep, or at the last ascent from sleep, may account for those strange mini-dream-like sensations, which characteristically occur during stage 1, NREM sleep, called hypnagogic or hypnapompic phenomena (depending on whether one is falling asleep or emerging from sleep).

THE USE OF DREAMS

But what of the "use" of dreams? Oracles, carnival barkers, analysts of every stripe, and, of course, the general public have all been fascinated by the prospect of knowing something from one's dreams. Let us, herewith, demystify the process of dream psychoanalysis. Dream analysis, unlike cocktail party hypnosis, does not often lend itself to spectacular guru-like pyrotechnics, much less to instantaneous curtain-raising revelations. Rather, it is quite literally a process of "analysis" . . . the steadfast attention to detail and historical context, and the application of such data to a current dream product presented within an interpersonal exchange between a dream narrator and a dream listener. For many, in addition to whatever other functions they may serve, dreams are meant to be communicated, and it is with the conveyance of the dream message to another that these particular dreamers bring their dreaming activity to a completion. Viewed in this light, the dreaming process is not much removed from the creative process in which an artistic product (be it a painting, poem, or play) must be communicated to a larger audience for the artist to feel that his work has been brought to completion.

It must be kept in mind that in psychoanalysis, when a patient reports a dream to the analyst, they are both engaged in an intensive interaction in which the relationship itself is the microscope's stage upon which the behavior patterns to be analyzed are being acted out and scrutinized, and within which subtle issues such as parent–child authority conflicts, the wish to please, and the need to resist or reveal may be resurrected from the patient's past and re-enacted in the present. So the dreamer tells his or her dream and the psychoanalyst listens. In this context, dreams are used by the listener as a source of information regarding the mental workings of the individual that provide diagnostic clues to underlying personality concerns. For, although modern psycho-analysts recognize the biochemical and neurophysiological subs-trate upon which the phenomenon of dreaming occurs, no one as yet has any biological explanation and understanding of individ-ual dreams. For this, we have to turn to psychology and the metaphors of behavior.

Freud enumerated the processes by which an analyst might approach a reported dream and how he might ultimately "inter-pret" it. First of all, the analyst would listen to the dream; listen to the thoughts and feelings the dreamer expressed and reflected around the report of the dream. He . . . incidentally, lest I be accused of being the same sexist, chauvinist that Freud has been, I use "he" out of convenience, not as the generic term for person-hood . . . he might ask the dreamer about associated events of the previous day or for a report of the chronological associations paralleling the dream story. He might ask the dreamer to "associ-ate to" a particularly striking image in the dream. Whatever would be done would be directed by the analyst's intimate knowledge of the dreamer's style of thinking and problem-solving, world view, underlying needs and concerns, and intercurrent life events as well as past history comprising the individual's memory store. As Charles Brenner writes (1969), "The decision as to what was appropriate and useful to interpret at the time is determined by factors other than the dream interpretation proper . . ." That is, the interpretation of dreams cannot be done by rote procedure, cookbook-fashion. Books purporting to give a pat formulary of dream symbols and interpretations, claiming universal appli-cability to all, may be of interest to read but are of relatively limited use.

In that same paper, Brenner goes on to say that in utilizing a dream presented by a patient and interpreting its meaning, as well as conveying this interpretation to the patient, "one is influenced by the previous course of the patient's analysis, by one's knowledge of what has already been interpreted to him, how he has re-sponded to previous interpretations, the state of the transference, the general level of resistance, one's knowledge of special events that may be upsetting . . ." The latter considerations (too involved for a simple explication here) notwithstanding, the point is that the process of dream interpretation in an exploratory and therapeutic context is an involved and many-faceted procedure, not a sideshow exhibit or a sleight-of-hand performance.

So what does the analyst do? How does he organize his thinking when confronted with the dreamer's dream? Brenner summarizes some of the procedures nicely. First, the analyst recognizes that dreams, like many behavioral symptoms, are perceived by individuals as odd, not really "belonging" to them. The term "ego alien" is used by psychiatrists to describe this phenomenon. He will recognize that although the majority of the content of the dream may be "disowned" by the dreamer, the emotion (or affect) associated with the dream has often retained a purity of relevance to the dreamer. That is why a dreamer may consciously be not only puzzled by the apparently bizarre dream story, but also confused by the vivid and moving emotions he experiences along with the relatively meaningless dream story. So the analyst is cognizant of the fact that the emotion accompanying the underlying content of the dream offers a relatively clear glimpse into the psychological meaning of the dream, to the dreamer, and remains the dream component least distorted by the particular form of thinking and processing that occurs in the dreaming process.

Secondly, he will work under the assumption that part of the reason that the dream content as remembered by the dreamer seems so strange and without apparent meaning is that cognitive functions like displacement, condensation, substitution, and representability (processes which Freud collected under the heading "dream work" and which are the creative and metaphorical cognitive functions of the dreamer) were in operation. A further assumption is that the task of these cognitive functions is to translate the latent content of a dream (perhaps arising from the imagistic memory stores in the right cerebral hemisphere) into a language (Freud's "primary process") and a resultant product . . . the manifest dream, or the dream as remembered and reported. Understanding that the dream end-product is the result of reworking accomplished by the cognitive functions associated with "dream work" (resulting in concealment of the original stimulus to the dream) and therefore in need of translation, the analyst may ask the dreamer for associations to the dream, which is **not** the same as asking what the patient what he or she thinks the dream means.

He will look, in the dream content, for evidences of psychological defenses which may serve as an impediment to eventual awareness of the underlying content. He may tentatively tie together the dream as presented with life events, in order to allay anxiety and proceed with the uncovering of more inapparent meaning. In doing this, he will have had to identify the theme of the manifest content of the dream, the significance of the style in which it is reported, and the pattern and sequence in which the dream components and associations arise. Finally, the psychoanalyst will attend to what the dreamer will consciously accept and act on, as a guide as to what he will accept in an interpretation.

Now let us return to the dream specimens with which this chapter opened and try to understand something of their meaning. I will supply enough information (while still protecting the anonymity of the dreamers) to supplement our brief glimpse, but keep in mind that we are in effect looking at "disembodied" dreams which only take on their full richness and poignant meaning when worked with in the context of interplay among dream, dreamer, and analyst.

Look back to the beginning of this chapter. The first dream is replete with associations to on-going issues in the dreamer's analysis. I will intersperse some of the dreamer's subsequent associations to the dream (in parentheses) in the retelling of it:

> I dreamt I was being led down a green corridor (I feel very green, new at this process . . . analysis . . . it also costs a lot! . . . green cash) to a green gas chamber (to gas is to talk, like in here), like Caryl Chessman (Carol, a woman's name . . . lying here on the couch makes me feel like less of a man than you . . . Chessman . . . wasn't he a rapist, taking advantage of helpless victims . . . Chess makes me think of strategy and game-playing). I knew the procedure, so I wasn't worried (any new procedure worries me). The executioner was talking to me through a mesh grating, like a microphone or a confessional (patient refers to similarities between his feelings toward his father and the analyst). He told me to hold my breath when I hear the pellet drop (recollections of early childhood and disciplinary struggles). But, suddenly, I panicked, fearing that maybe I didn't know the process as well as I thought I did, and I didn't want to die!

Briefly, this patient had a life-long history of trying to escape from anticipated condemnation by elders in authority, attempting to triumph through passivity (in his words: "by trying to be the **best** nice guy!"), but feeling always less of a man for it, with a sense that behind every turn there's something bad lurking. Successful resolution of his difficulties with asserting himself led to much more gratifying relationships with women as well.

Now, remember the second dream, with its allusions to self-examination and living plants. It is a beautiful, almost Zen-like, description of a young woman's sense of growth and courage as she approached the end of her analysis. Initially her response to the dream was that its feeling-tone was exceptionally meaningful and "personal" to her. But the actual images seemed silly and a little confusing to her. She ultimately responded to the whimsical nature of the content, a reflection of the charming whimsy that this woman was beginning to allow to flourish.

With regard to the third dream, it ultimately revealed to the dreamer his tremendous sense of betrayal and vulnerability (some analysts like to use the term "castration anxiety"!) following a disastrous love relationship. Exploration of the relationship, and this dream, triggered memories of problematic interactions with his mother from his earliest years. As his analysis progressed, increasingly greater inroads were made into the tortured and agony-filled private life he was leading, in many ways consciously unbeknownst even to him and manifested "only" by a persistent pattern of destructive love relationships, struggles with authority figures, and dissatisfaction with his career. Let me share with you an edited version of a dream from midway through this fellow's analysis during a time when he was experiencing much discomfort regarding continued analytic exploration of his sense of manhood (not, he felt, because he had some hidden homosexual conflict, but because he was "intellectually embarrassed" about "becoming a textbook caricature"). This dream illustrates the power of the visual, pictorial image and the emotional content that may be attached to it, and marked the beginning of an important chapter and a step forward in his analysis (again, the thoughts set off in parentheses are those the patient verbalized in association with the images of the dream):

> I was riding a motorcycle at night through rainy streets in a town with the lights reflecting off the street. The roadway was slippery (it was hazardous, like the nighttime slicked streets I've raced down in Europe). I went through the right-hand arch of a viaduct while

someone else on a motorcycle was coming through in the opposite
direction from the left-hand arch (it was a three-arched viaduct . . .
one large central arch and two smaller ones on either side . . . phallic
arches! . . . A viaduct carries water, and sewerage . . . water under
the bridge! . . . In that kind of situation, you're afraid of spinning
out . . . maybe afraid of that here too . . . I have a memory of a
magician with a black bag . . . what's up your sleeve?! It's you, and I'm
afraid you'll disappear . . . or maybe abandon me . . . I see myself
coming and going, taking action which is guaranteed to keep me in
the same place!).

A summary of Freud's dream theory is that dreams are the
mental representations of demanding but forbidden wishes. Because of the prohibitions against its fulfillment (for instance because it derives from infantile impulses for immediate and, in the
adult world of decorous civility, unseemly satisfaction), the wish is
distorted and reworked through the dreaming process until its
original intent is disguised sufficiently through cognitive mechanisms such as symbolization and condensation. In other words, a
taboo thought or urge is censored and replaced with a more
acceptable mental representation, which still, however, retains
some connection to the underlying forbidden wish. It follows then
that this link is potentially discoverable through the processes of
psychoanalysis, using free association, in particular.

As previously discussed, McCarley and Hobson disagree that
the instigator of the dream is the forbidden wish. They hold that
the instigators are the amoral, unthinking, unfeeling pontine
brainstem cells driven by a cyclical chronobiological mandate to
fire up every 90 minutes or so during sleep. Others, too, may differ
with the original Freudian formulation and may do so not by
jumping psychological ship to physiological freighter, but by arguing, still within a psychological framework, that the process of
dreaming may not be as idiosyncratic, haphazard and catch-as-
catch-can as the Freudian model might suggest, and, furthermore, by pointing out that there is a difference between the
psychoanalytic *theory* of dream formation and the *process* of dream
interpretation. The caricature of the overly intellectualized dream
unscrambling, often found in popular magazine articles, is **not**
psychoanalysis. Dream interpretation, when done (and often, it
should be noted, the dream is of more use to the analyst as a
monitor of the patient's progress rather than as a vehicle for

interpreting behavior), preferably springs from the dreamer's associations, even though the dreamer reports a dream and may then demand "Alright, Doc, what does it mean?!"

There is a similarity between the dream-interpreting techniques of the psychoanalyst and the techniques of the descriptive anthropologist. Both use a naturalistic approach in which the subject informs the investigator about his own experience and the investigator listens to how the subject talks about his experience. From the very use of language, the subject is thought to reveal information about, first, his own language structure, and second, the thought processes and personality characteristics underlying the language descriptions.

Language is one of the basic tools of behavioral scientists who deal with humans. They use language to elicit verbal behavior from patients which, in turn, is analyzed to understand the enduring determinants of behavior, known as personality. Language is also used as a therapeutic tool to modify behavior. Eliciting and analyzing language patterns is therefore seen as a primary, although not exclusive, source of data providing a window into the psychological realm of experiential action and reaction, the significance of which the individual may not have fully appreciated. The analyst takes this one step further and attempts not only to dig like the archeologist for what have been called "artifacts of the mind" (i.e., dreams), but to use the language of the dream as a reflecting mirror of the individual's picture of his/her continuity of identity, and also to teach the individual to begin to listen more appreciatively to the subtle whispers of the brain in his/her ear during sleep.

And what about kids? They dream too. David Foulkes published a book in 1982 entitled *Children's Dreams: Longitudinal Studies* in which he chronicled the developmental change in dream characteristics paralleling a child's growth and accompanying cognitive development. He noted that, in early childhood, dreams were simple, relatively mundane and not, contrary to what many had thought, filled with rich, frightening fairy tale-like imagery. He reported that by the ages of 7–9 years, kids begin to have more extended and more detailed narratives with some motivation assigned to the dream characters. Within the next two years, in general, young dreamers appear in their own dreams for the first time as major characters. An additional finding of interest reported by Foulkes was that the presence of daytime anxiety in these children functioned more as a wet blanket than as a stimulus to more vivid and elaborate dreams.

However these data are eventually understood and integrated into the larger body of sleep-related knowledge, it is generally felt, from the subjective point of view of the adult dreamer, that the dream provides a "virtual" reality, weaving tapestries from the filaments of life's events . . . like viewing an Edward Hopper painting in which you are halfway in the painting and halfway outside it.

> Once upon a time I, Chuang Tzu, dreamt I was a butterfly . . .
> following my fancies unconscious of my individuality as a man . . .
> Now I do not know whether I was a man dreaming I was a butterfly
> or whether I am now a butterfly dreaming I am a man . . . It is only at
> the great awakening that one knows that all has only been a dream.
> *Chuang Tzu, Book II*, Chi-Chen Wang translation cited in Martin
> S. Bergmann, 1966.

It is easy to understand how, in the initial stages of dream exploration, this state was viewed as a temporary psychosis by some, where the hallucinatory type of activity, along with the bizarre thoughts and reasoning, suggested the interchangeability of schizophrenic and REM mentation to some who ultimately concluded that schizophrenia represented an intrusion of the REM state into wakefulness. However, neither was this conclusion supported by subsequent investigation, nor was it found that the REM state is abnormal in schizophrenia. The two phenomena do not appear to be related in any significant functional way.

MIND AND BRAIN, DREAMS AND REM SLEEP

Which theory most closely accounts for the business of dreaming, whether it be one that attributes a purposeful brain function to dreaming (such as a "recharging" function or a perhaps a "tonic-stimulating" one), or one which holds that dreaming is the consequence of an inherent quality of the brain, surfacing during certain shifts in states of arousal, remains to be seen. Support for this latter consideration (that dreaming is an inherent activity of the brain because any organ so configured neuro-physiologically would, by definition, behave that way . . . that is, a characteristic-of-the-organ kind of reasoning) goes back to some of the isolation tank experiments of Dr. John Lilly done in the 1950s in which volunteers, suspended in a neutral environment devoid of all external stimuli, began to experience while awake, vivid and florid perceptual experiences with the characteristics of dream-like hallucinations. Something about the removal of external stimuli seemed to allow the waking brain's natural propensity to create its own hallucinatory reality to come to the surface, if left to its own devices.

This is but one aspect of the biological nature of that organ of the mind, the brain, which will require much further understanding in order to shed light on the nature of the dreaming process and the possible functions served by its products. Another issue that must await further clarification involves the status and significance of dreams outside of the REM state. Whether the occurrence, or at least harvesting, of vivid dreams during NREM sleep, for instance, negates the general tenet of the activation-synthesis hypothesis of McCarley and Hobson is, in one sense, beside the point.

It is important to remember that there may be quite a significant difference between what stimulates a dream to be initiated, what factors then determine how the tale is spun out, and what mechanisms are called into play to enhance the elaboration, recall and recounting of the dream. An entire group of procedures involved with information processing and communication is called into play, only one of which may involve the differential functioning of the two cerebral hemispheres or the cyclical firing of sleep pacemaker cells deep within the brainstem. It also remains to be seen whether certain biological components are the necessary and sufficient constituents of an explanation of certain psychological states. The task that all serious investigators have wrestled with is that of melding psychic phenomena and biological mechanisms into one unified and coherent theory of understanding. And they continue to do so, for one cannot make casual inferences between disparate classes—whether they be understanding the events, the processes of sensation and perception, the nature of memory, or the essence of sleep and dreaming—one needs an "umbrella"

category encompassing them all, in order to make these connections. In other words, there must be, to mix a metaphor or two,
many ways for our "blind men," in Chapter 4, to skin a cat . . . with
all due apologies to animal lovers.

Early psychoanalytic thinkers considered dreaming either as
an attempt, using camouflage, to allow erupting but forbidden
infantile wishes to be fulfilled and thereby calm the individual
(Freud), as a safety valve to allow for blowing off steam generated
by overreactions during the previous day (Jung), or as an opportunity to rehearse the next day's activities (Adler). Perhaps these
formulations, in light of our current knowledge, represent more
poetry than science, but poetry, too, can yield information for us.
Whether we choose to replace Freud's universal categories of
sexuality, forbidden impulses, and so forth, with a different set of
universal categories based in the language of what is currently
known in the neurosciences . . . whether we view the dream as a
created script disguising an underlying knowable personality
dynamic, or as the test pattern generated by a brain retooling and
returning itself for the next period of arousal . . . it should be
remembered that dreaming does reflect a way of thinking, and
further, that in many instances, thought can be a dress rehearsal
for action.

So the next time someone at a cocktail party gives you a one-
sentence report and then asks you, from your newfound fount of
information, to interpret his or her dream, be mindful of several
things. First, that the dream phenomenon is a psychological concomitant of a biological perturbation during sleep; second, that
the sharing of dreams and request for understanding have communicative importance in their own right, whether the subject
matter shared or interpreted is a public product or a more private
one. Finally, remember that catch phrases regarding so-called
universal themes in dreams can mean little about a specific dream
or its specific meaning to a given individual . . . although they **can**
keep the conversational momentum going!

Just as it would seem obvious that the complexity and organization of dreams is dependent on cognitive capacities such as the
ability to abstract, or to use symbolic and visual representations for
verbal fabrications, so too it should be appreciated that differences
between individuals, regarding these same functions, will deter-

mine different qualities of the dreams which are reported. As such, the dream becomes a mirror reflecting qualities of personality, temperament, and previous history that help to delineate the individual and differentiate him from his fellowmen. This is so, regardless of what is considered to be the energizing source (psychological or biological) of the dream fountain. It is certainly time for the (new) biological psychologists to stop beating a dead (Freudian) horse. Freud's initial attribution to dreams, of a mechanistic and sleep-preserving function in an arena in which ferocious internal instincts vie with societally prescribed repressions for supremacy, was an initial, and brilliant, attempt to codify a psychology of dreams and dreaming using the data available at the time. We know more now, and we stand on the threshold of an entirely new and expanded appreciation of the workings of the mind, within the brain. However, it is still generally accepted that whatever the source of the emotional currents and memory shards that accumulate under the rubric of a particular dream, this conglomeration is reworked into a larger, more completed tapestry, the dream as reported, and, as such, represents a repository of much personal relevance and meaning to the individual dreamer. Whether or not some of this "*post hoc*" editorial work on the dream is meant to obscure some underlying significance and to distract the dreamer from the latent conflicts hidden within, it is most likely that when the virtuous person states "I would never dream of such a thing!" he is probably correct . . . under ordinary circumstances!

Chapter 9

Ondine's Curse—and Other Sleeping Sicknesses

> The water nymph, Ondine, even though an immortal, was
> smitten by an ordinary bloke, a knight, and married him. He,
> however, did not remain faithful to her. The enraged nymph
> took her revenge . . . by cursing him with death if he were ever
> to sleep.

The "central hypoventilation syndrome," or "Ondine's curse," was
first recognized in the mid 1950's. It is a disorder which does not
exist during waking hours, while conscious control over breathing
patterns holds sway. Instead, it appears that with sleep, or the loss
of consciousness, the breathing that we all take for granted does
not continue, presumably because of a faulty element in the
automatic, nonconscious breathing control mechanisms that reside in the brainstem. Sufferers of "Ondine's curse" "forget" to
breathe, so to speak, when they sleep. The neurological "automatic
pilot," which is supposed to take over control of respiration during
sleep, does not respond to the oxygen needs of the body. Normally,
much of the brain can sleep while select centers of nervous activity,
like night watchmen in a power generating plant watch, adjust and
fine-tune activities according to the maintenance needs of the
system. But in the individual with Ondine's curse, the night
watchman sleeps too. Usually, the syndrome can be identified
within a few hours of birth, when the affected child takes on a
peculiar bluish tinge, known as cyanosis (a reflection of poor

oxygenation of the blood), and exhibits periods of greatly reduced if not totally absent respiratory movements during periods of slumber. Not to be confused with voluntary breath-holding of the 1- or 2-year old, or the swimmer's suppression of his breathing by voluntary hyperventilation just prior to diving underwater, "Ondine's curse" refers to a deficiency in the brain's control of automatic breathing—in other words, a defect in the central control mechanisms of breathing.

We have already established that sleep is **not** a passive "nonstate." It is **not** a mere hiatus in the activity cycles of "real" living, allowing the sleeper to just bide his or her time until he or she can rejoin the mainstream of life. Sleep, although it is time-out from one set of activities, is not dead time. Sleep is an active process, with complex neurochemical systems interwoven and alternately ascending and descending in dominance—with the adrenalin system predominating during the cycles of REM sleep, and with acetylcholine and its "parasympathetic" system dominating during NREM sleep. Coupled with the intricate orchestration of various brain chemical systems and neurological pacemakers which direct the nature and characteristics of the sleep cycle, are factors such as the individual's age, general state of health, external environmental stresses, and circumstances which also affect the characteristics of sleep, like its overall duration as well as the amount of time spent in each of the different sleep stages. Sleeping, like eating and other general functions of living, can affect and be affected by the general state of bodily well-being. As an example, studies are increasingly demonstrating a significant interconnection between the immune system and sleep. For instance, a number of naturally occurring chemicals called neuropeptides, with specific names such as factor S, muramyl peptides, alpha interferon, and interleukin-1, which help to govern the body's immunological defense response to disease invaders, also facilitate sleep. Although, as we have previously discussed, a presumed restorative function for sleep (allowing for body repair of the wear and tear visited upon it during waking activity) has not been established, the facts that (1) the agents listed above affect both immunological responses and sleep, and (2) during sleep, changes occur in the activity of disease-fighting cells (like blood lymphocytes and the shock-troops going under the rather fearsome name of natural killer cells, or NKs), suggests that aspects of the metabolic function of cells are altered with sleep, and perhaps with sleep loss.

But sleep, being a dynamic process with many different elements, can also suffer disorders of its own inherent function. And it is to the disorders of sleep that we now turn our attention.

> Rip Van Winkle is awakened by his wife after his long hibernation, so the joke goes. "Rip, Rip! Wake up! You've been asleep for 20 years!" she said. Turning away, while trying to burrow his head, he allegedly replied "Aw . . . just give me ten more minutes." Here we have another sleep curiosity, dubbed the Rip Van Winkle Syndrome, after Washington Irving's description of irresistible sleepiness, disorientation, forgetfulness, and confusion that overcame the legendary Van Winkle and allowed him to wonder that his 20-year sleep ". . . had been to him but as one night . . ." That, in the innermost landscape of the Catskill mountains. Here, in the halls of medicine, we are less puzzled by this phenomenon, and, unlike "Ondine's curse," the causative event is well-understood. Here the discrete compromise of blood supply to select areas of the brain following a cerebrovascular accident (or "small stroke") is the culprit, not some fabled goblins' brew. Nor is this the only example of the obverse of the aphorism that "life imitates art."

◆   ◆   ◆

> The obese boy, Joe, of Charles Dickens's *The Posthumous Papers of the Pickwick Club*, or the giant in *Jack and the Beanstalk* both serve as models of the individual whose respirations are physically restricted because of obesity and who, therefore, suffer from decreased breathing (called "hypoventilation") and sleeping bouts jerkily disrupted and interspersed with waking sleepiness. Here we see portrayed characteristics of the individual with obstructive sleep apnea—a physiological dysfunction of respiration occurring during sleep resulting in some form of airway obstruction, snoring, disrupted sleep, and consequent daytime sleepiness. A bevy of fairytale beauties, such as Snow White (poisoned by a drug-laced apple), Sleeping Beauty (stuck by a contaminated sewing needle), or The Princess (of "The Princess and the Pea" fame . . . tossing and turning in bed at night), further support the notion that, when it comes to sleep, art "imitates" life!

Disorders of sleep, and certainly complaints about sleep, are prominent phenomena and, like other common conditions, can derive from many different causes and can display a broad range of manifestations. From the fussing infant to the pacing elderly adult; from the "stressed-out" college sophomore to the late-shift worker; from the depressed widow to the jet-lagged business traveler—all can suffer some form of sleep disruption. In fact, current evidence indicates that a minimum of one-third of adults, at any one time, complain of insomnia. Since sleeplessness seems to be such a prevalent complaint, and can be a symptom representing responses to many varied and different medical, psychological, and situational problems and circumstances, it is essential to identify the significant factors that provide clues to the underlying problem. It does no good to focus solely on the symptom whose existence may merely be a reflection of the far larger, base problem lying underneath, any more than it does to focus only on that floating pyramidal tip which represents only a small portion of the iceberg dwelling beneath the surface of Arctic seas. The clinician must be like the Northern Sea ship's captain, alert, seeking clues and not lulled into inattention toward less apparent processes also going on. Curiously, patients themselves may not always be of the best help here. Hurting from the discomfort, for instance, of sleep deprivation, they may identify the insomnia as their primary problem and balk at the physician who opts for the slower, ostensibly less direct route of diagnostic evaluation before resorting to the longed-for "magic bullet" . . . the sleeping pill.

Sleep disorders may be classified not just according to the complaints of light or fragmented sleep patterns. They may be organized into categories relating to age, to the presence of accompanying medical or environmental conditions, and to the very nature of the specific sleep phase affected (and in what way). Although much of this "cataloging," particularly in the early stages of any scientific accumulation of knowledge, can seem like fussing between great uncertainty and talmudic splitting-of-hairs, it is not. The attempt to find unifying principles of anatomic, chemical, physiological, or behavioral activity, and then to be able to subtype different functional derangements of the sleep process in terms of these, allows us to not only direct ourselves to more appropriate treatment strategies, but also to continue in a systematic exploration of the very nature of the sleep process itself. The hallmarks of any emerging medical discipline, therefore, appear as a "nosology"—a cataloging of diseases and syndromes, along with their accompanying symptoms and signs.

Although caffeine is reportedly used by up to 80 percent of the adult population with impugnity, the pharmacologic effects of caffeine at dose ranges found in two cups of coffee (160–180 milligrams), can worsen preexisting anxiety and depression, can interfere with the onset of sleep and, with some, contrary to what one might anticipate, can lead to early morning drowsiness. This last effect may be because caffeine subtly disrupted the previous night's rest, or because caffeine withdrawal overnight culminates in morning sedation. As with any pharmacologic agent, there may be a wide range of individual sensitivities, accounting for one man's meat being another's poison. In addition, there are powerful psychological forces that work in conjunction with the pharmacological effects to determine a particular agent's affect on a particular individual, at a particular time. Such forces account for the important and pervasive "placebo effect." But, on average, it would take a massive dose of caffeine (two to four cups of coffee) at bedtime to create significant fragmentation of sleep. Smaller effects, of course, can occur with smaller "doses," and we always have to make adequate allowance for that elusive factor, "individual differences."

With regard to the functional disturbances of sleep, clinicians must consider in addition to, say, differences between children and the aged, the possible contributions of differing personality types to sleep processes, and the possibility that other contributing, or at least confounding, conditions may be operating which can create a more generalized disorganization or dyscontrol of body rhythm synchronization. For any symptom, be it sleep disturbance or personality quirk, could represent an attempt by the individual to organize around some subtle biologically based dyscontrol, as well as being a more direct expression and consequence of the dyscontrol itself.

On a less theoretical level, we are developing a more sophisticated armamentarium with which to deal with sleep disorders. This includes treatments for certain medical illnesses, the education of individuals regarding sleep needs, characteristics and practices, the correct use of hypnotic agents and psychotropic medications, and the effective use of psychological interventions like psychotherapy and the behavioral therapies. But all are predicated on diagnosis—understanding what pathological phenomena may be related and, by virtue of some commonality of underlying cause, may be responsive to a particular therapeutic endeavor.

Since just about everybody, at one time or another, has trouble sleeping, and since there is no such thing as a "quick fix" for a symptom like insomnia, which can arise from many different antecedents (acting alone or in varying degrees of concert), it is important for anyone, sufferer or treater, to evaluate, first off, the individual's sleep complaint and not jump too soon in either the direction of summary reassurance or the path of the soporific bandwagon.

Let us take a brief example. First of all, we assume (1) that the functioning and productions of the brain are purposeful whether we are awake or asleep (only, perhaps, they manifest their meaning differently in these different states), and (2) that the maintenance of vital life functions like respiration and circulation remains under central nervous system control whether we are awake or asleep—thank goodness we have one less thing to worry about! In other words, we take for granted that our varying states of activation/alertness interplay intimately with other aspects of physiological functioning. Therefore, since disturbances of sleep may bring physiological consequences to the individual, all complaints of chronic poor sleep must be evaluated with care. Not all sleep complaints are necessarily associated with either psychological and social problems, or with anxiety, depression, and certain personality traits (like aggression and compulsion). Although these factors can be primary, so too can be disturbances in the sleep process itself. Up to 50 percent of insomnia is related to psychiatric problems or what is loosely called "stress," while 10-15 percent is associated with drug or alcohol use and abuse. This leaves about 35 percent of cases founded in organic neurological and other medically related problems. It follows that, just for this reason alone, it is important to search for the specific underlying cause of any sleep complaint. Additionally, it is generally felt that with acute distress, and its concomitant short-term insomnia, treatment differs from that accompanying either a more profound situational traumatic event or the whole panoply of medical, psychiatric and environmental problems supporting more long-standing sleep disruptions.

To return to our now no longer brief aside. Recently some public acclaim has been given to longitudinal studies suggesting that there is a connection between longevity and the average length of nightly sleep. It was reported that both extremes, the "meager" sleeper (getting 4 hours or less every night) and the "excessive" sleeper (regularly sleeping 10 or more hours nightly) have a life expectancy one-half that of their contemporaries, who sleep more in the middle range. These reported statistics, first, add modern-day attention-getting drama to the observation of Hippocrates, 400 years B.C., that "Sleep and watchfulness, both of these when immoderate, constitute disease." But, secondly, they (plus the commonplace phenomenon of the sleepiness complaint itself) are used to fill popular magazines with claims of a pervasive state of sleep deprivation for most of us.

But let us consider what these reports really indicate. They could, of course, mean that in fact sleep complaints and increased mortality are directly related. But what about the underlying disorders that may be causing the sleep complaints to begin with? Is there a difference, with regard to mortality, between narcolepsy and a brain tumor, both of which can cause excessive daytime sleepiness and can be associated with increased mortality (through accidents in the former, and through terminal compromise of neurological function in the latter)? Is there a difference with regard to shift work and sleep apnea? Furthermore, do the micro-awakenings of sleep apnea contribute to mortality at all, and, if so, do they do it in some way directly or indirectly via effects on personality, mood and general health? The vast majority of shift workers, whose schedules constantly change, complain of insomnia, daytime fatigue, stomach problems, and family problems. But what are the characteristics of those workers who have "survived" years of constant shift work? These individuals form a small but significant group who apparently show none of the above-mentioned symptoms. Here we may be dealing with the question of "stress" (the necessary concomitant of life) and the effect of "distress" (the unsatisfactory adaptation to stress) on morbidity and mortality.

The point is that there are many factors that must be taken into account when evaluating definitive claims such as the one with which this "brief aside" began. It is certainly possible that sleep duration may ultimately prove to have some statistical correlation with mortality rates. However, we must also remember that sleep itself may be a behavioral "epiphenomenon," fascinating in and of itself, but distracting our attention from the confluens of biological and chemical processes far below which are affecting not only measures of the sleep cycle itself but also of culminating events such as death.

> Count Dracula languishes in his coffin, waiting for the stroke of midnight so that he may be released. The clock strikes twelve but, lo, at first he cannot move. All we see is the flicker of eyes darting back and forth. The paralysis during his transition into alertness has yet to dissipate. And another model of a phenomenon of sleep—in which the individual feels unable to move or to speak and which may be associated with a sense of heaviness on the chest, and hallucinatory experiences—is committed to literary immortality.
>
> Examples of isolated sleep paralysis attacks (so called because they are not associated with any other sleep disorder, like narcolepsy) can occur in people who are in all other ways ostensibly healthy. It is found in other cultures as well and is called, quaintly enough, "Old Hag" in rural Canada, *Kanashibari* in Japan (referring to the gods of Buddhism) and *kokma* in the Caribbean islands—all of which incorporate the idea of a "possession" creating temporary paralysis. Thought by some investigators now to represent an inherited trait, sleep paralysis tends to be considered an example of physiological abnormality rather than pathology in need of specific treatment other than education and reassurance.

THE SPECTRUM OF SLEEP DISORDERS

The following outline will provide us with an overview of disorders of sleep so that we may first more systematically discuss them and then, subsequently, methodically turn our attention to treatment options. However, in any healthy and dynamic, multi-disciplinary science that is growing, there will be a number of different perspectives possible. For instance, in 1979, the Association of Sleep Disorders Centers established diagnostic criteria based heavily on the characteristic patterns of the sleep-EEG. The resulting classification divided sleep disorders into the following categories: disorders of initiating and maintaining sleep (DIMS), that is, the insomnias; disorders of excessive somnolence (DOES); disorders of the sleep–wake schedule (brought on, for example, by stimulant or sedative use or by a misalliance between an individual's sleep–wake cycle and the demands of his/her environment); and parasomnias (disorders that are not actual disturbances in sleep itself, but occur exclusively in and around sleep, and therefore can interfere with sleep, or are made worse by the sleeping state). These categories are not mutually exclusive, however (since DIMS and DOES can coexist in many conditions), and many clinical situations do not lend themselves to simple assignment in one category to the exclusion of the others.

Another classification of sleep disorders, that of the American Psychiatric Association's *DSM-III-R* is symptom-focused: all disorders are divided into the dyssomnias (in which the amount, quality, or timing of sleep is disordered) and the parasomnias (in which abnormal events occur during sleep or during the transition between sleep and wakefulness). For our purposes, we will look at an amalgam of the classification systems, keeping in mind that the particular effects of age and aging may account for specific sleep disorder phenomena outside the scope of the following schema.

As a general outline, consider the following:

1. Insomnia (transient or chronic):
   a. Physiologic (naturally occurring with age)
   b. Primary, or delayed-sleep phase syndrome
   c. Secondary to: sleep-related respiratory disorders (apnea); sleep-related movement disorders; psychological states (depression, anxiety, "conditioned" insomnia); environmental disruption and/or discomfort; medical disorders causing pain, itch or cramps; pregnancy; drug and alcohol use or withdrawal; medical disorders (such as asthma, ulcer disease, thyroid disease, hypoglycemia, coronary artery disease, urological disorders, and neurological syndromes)
2. Hypersomnia (transient or chronic):
   a. Physiologic
   b. Primary or "idiopathic"
   c. Secondary to: sleep-related respiratory disorders; sleep-related movement disorders; narcolepsy; psychological states (seasonal affective disorder, atypical depression, anxiety); environmental disruption, discomfort or demands (work shift, jet lag); menstrually related conditions; drug and alcohol use; obesity; medical disorders (such as epilepsy, toxic exposure to lead, head trauma, thyroid disease, liver disease, encephalitis, syphilis, and

two unusual syndromes—one, a rare, self-limited disorder of young males who may exhibit irritability and
aggressive behavior along with sleepiness, over-eating,
and hypersexuality, called the Kleine-Levin syndrome;
the other, an unusual neurological condition involving
the intrusion of EEG-alpha wave activity, which is normally associated with a drowsy waking state, into stages
of deep sleep, and associated with complaints of sleepiness, chronic fatigue, muscle aches and eating disorders)
3. Dyssomnias: Sleepwalking (somnambulism) and sleep
talking (somniloquy); night terrors (*pavor nocturnus*); bedwetting (enuresis); teeth-grinding (bruxism); head-banging;
excessive snoring; sleep-related cluster headaches; other
sleep-related movement disorders

The above outline is just meant to give an overview of the range
and scope of disorders of sleep and disorders during sleep. It is
a schematic chart, not a definitive atlas of the landscape of sleep-
related disorders.

About half of all patients referred to sleep laboratory centers
will have a chief complaint of daytime sleepiness and will be
diagnosed as having a DOES. Thirty percent will complain of a
DIMS . . . this according to Drs. Roffwarg and Erman, who
summarized their findings in the *1985 APA Annual Review*. With
regard to insomnia, once chronic, it can be described irrespective
of its initiating or triggering circumstance. It seems that with the
passage of time most long-term insomniacs become as one in
terms of their psychology and the expression of concern about
sleep. Anxious ruminations and presleep mullings are characteristic of many if not all people with chronic complaints of poor sleep.
Studies by Drs. Joyce and Anthony Kales and co-workers at the
Sleep Research and Treatment Center of the Penn State University College of Medicine (1987) revealed characteristic feelings of
mental fatigue, "mind racing," and "difficulty relaxing" in insomniacs, as well as an abundance of activities such as bedtime
reading, eating, drinking (including alcoholic beverages), and
going to the bathroom as compared with non-insomniacs. What
does **not** distinguish those with sleep problems from those without
them is the desire for the amount of sleep. Interestingly, insomniacs do not seem to long for undue amounts of sleep. It is only

that they find getting **any** restful and satisfying slumber elusive. Whether it is difficulty getting to sleep, problems staying asleep, disruptive early morning awakening, or a general sense of having slept unsatisfactorily, the insomniac, regardless of the underlying etiology of the insomnia, often has generalized negative associations with sleep, and many of these attitudes carry over into daytime activities. One can well imagine, as we have all experienced to some extent, the dampening effect on physical and mental activities and social interactions of a sustained focus on a basically unsatisfactory one-third portion of one's life! Under these circumstances, the very act of trying to go to sleep produces anxiety and arousal of such proportions that the soft-spoken sleep-promoting mechanism may be overwhelmed. Or the sleeping environment takes on such noxious qualities for the insomniac that sleep cannot intervene. This is what is meant by "conditioned insomnia" listed under DIMS, above. Like Pavlov's dogs conditioned to respond by salivating to the ringing of a bell instead of to the actual presence of food, these individuals respond to certain sleep-associated cues with insomnia rather than with slumber. This particular form of insomnia is not limited to any age group. It can become established initially around some traumatic event and become so ingrained that the sleep problem persists long after the initial, precipitating conditions have passed. Because these people have become conditioned to the bedtime situation in a negative way, they can often find it easier to sleep away from familiar surrounds, or when they are not specifically trying to go to sleep. These people can often be seen asleep with the light on, the book open, and the TV on. In addition, they more often than not have a history of poor sleeping habits, including watching the clock with apprehension, having erratic hours for bedtime, late night eating, or working in bed.

Of course there are certain psychiatric disturbances which have direct effects on sleep, like anxiety (following a traumatic life event like a family move, a divorce, a job loss, or a death), or depression (with an extended time needed for sleep to begin, a decrease in total sleep time, increased number of middle-of-the-night awakenings, and difficulty getting up in the morning), and which are frequently associated with insomnia. Add to this list, in the elderly (whom we will discuss more, below), the presence of an organic mental syndrome (called dementia) with confusion and maybe agitation at night accounting for significant insomnia. This last case is essential to identify clearly because, if such a person is mistakenly treated with hypnotic sedative medication, this "sundowning" effect actually worsens (see below).

> Called *bangungut* among Philippine men or *pokkura* among Japanese men, the sudden, unexplained nocturnal death syndrome (SUNDS) has been reported in previously healthy young men, including Southeast Asian immigrants to the United States. Whether or not it is a unitary phenomenon and what its cause might be are both unknown at this point.

◆   ◆   ◆

> Sleep panic attacks are episodes of frightful dread which occur during the transition between sleep and arousal. They typically are associated with the various symptoms of daytime panics (heart palpitations, shortness of breath, flushing, perspiring), and can come on with relaxation, with sleep deprivation and/or with awakening. If one awakens with a panic attack, there is almost never any specific dream recollection. They, however, can also occur with relaxation and with sleep deprivation. So, for the sufferer of sleep panic attacks, there is a "catch-22": if, for fear of going to sleep and having an attack, one stays up, he incurs sleep deprivation and increases the likelihood of triggering the very attack that he was trying to avoid!

With regard to the environmental contribution to DIMS, certainly the physical characteristics of the sleeping environment play a role. Whether it is noise, temperature, light, the timing of eating and drinking, the familiarity of the surroundings, or even the softness of the mattress, physical attributes surrounding the sleep event can contribute to determining the quality of the experience. And so too can the internal environment in the sense that underlying medical and neurological disorders can have profound effects on sleep.

Sleep regulation occurs in the brain, as do certain other fucntions susceptible to alterations caused by neurological disturbances. As such, it is not surprising that they may all, on occasion, overlap, presenting us with an admixture of sleep disorders and neurological symptoms and signs based on specific diseases of the central nervous system. These include inflammation of the brain, known as encephalitis (the progressive mental lethargy, known as "sleeping sickness," caused by an infection by the organism *Trypanosoma gambiense*, transmitted to people in the tropics by the dreaded tsetse fly), or structural brain changes with accompanying disorganization of neurological function, whether generalized or discrete, caused by trauma, space-occupying tumor growth, or the decreased nurturing circulation of arteriosclerotic vascular disease. With many of these diseases there may be an initial disruption of sleep patterns but, as the destructive process advances, states of hypersomnolence—the sleeping part of "sleeping sickness," becomes more prominent. This increase in somnolence does not, however, represent an increase, or at times even a preponderance, of normal sleep architecture. Gradually, the distinct patterns, recognized on the EEG tracing and which, in the normal state, differentiate the particular stages of sleep, become more diffuse with indications of increasingly more odd brain electrical activity becoming more apparent. Additionally, there are degenerative diseases of the nervous system, diseases seemingly under the control of a genetic time-triggered "switch," with names ranging from the more familiar Parkinson's and Huntington's diseases, to the less familiar Shy-Drager syndrome or Ramsay Hunt syndrome. And of course there is the spectrum of disorders of brain electrical discharge, known as epileptic disorders, which may also present with sleep-related symptomatology.

It may seem obvious, from our image of the punch-drunk ex-prize fighter, that head trauma may lead to damage of neurological structures, disruption of their function, and interruption of normal sleep patterns. It may be less apparent, although no less certain, that various metabolic diseases and general systemic diseases (involving distant organs like the liver or kidneys), as well as intoxications and "toxications" (from chemicals as diverse as the metals manganese and lead, to the stimulants caffeine, theophyllin, and amphetamine) can affect sleep both quantitatively (from excessive sleepiness to morbid wakefulness) and qualitatively (with shifts in and disintegration of sleep architecture).

With regard to the interplay between other organ systems and sleep, most are involved. The well-known association of languid somnolence in big cats following the feast of a big kill, or the soporific effect of that big Thanksgiving meal in humans are well known and suggestive of the close relationship between the digestive system and sleep. Theories postulating important linkages between the functioning of the gastrointestinal system and sleep focus on the contribution of factors like (1) cholecystokinin, a naturally occurring agent with effects both in the head and the gut, (2) patterns of gastric acid secretion, with timed rhythmical swings (like those occurring with body temperature and the secretion of adrenalin and certain other neurotransmitters), from 2:00 PM highs to 2:00 AM lows, (3) patterns of intestinal motility (witness the nighttime flare-ups of diarrhea with some who suffer from diabetes or severe intestinal tract inflammatory disease), and (4) patterns of diurnal sensitivity to pain perception (with nocturnal heartburn from esophageal irritation and inflammation leading to complaints ranging from nighttime choking to chest pain).

> High altitude mountain climbers evidence disrupted sleep patterns. Whether this is due to a primary effect of altitude on sleep mechanisms, or is a secondary effect of a disruption of breathing during sleep (which has been documented) is as yet uncertain. But certainly some underlying mechanism, sensitive to the level of oxygen in the blood, seems to be affected. The cut-off point appears to be at about 12,000 feet; above this altitude, everyone can expect to experience difficulty falling asleep and staying asleep. Of course, the additional rigors of the climb itself, of the elevated level of arousal in general associated with the activity, and of time changes (particularly if traveling eastward) associated with a new and exotic locale can all contribute as well to sleep disruption.

COMPLAINTS OF INSUFFICIENT SLEEP

With the prominence of insomnia as a complaint and with the almost universal experience of it at one time or another in everyone's life, it is not surprising that some enterprising observers of the current scene have published claims that many of us, maybe even the vast majority, are sleep-deprived. This is a very serious "charge," with significant health, safety, and economic consequences and, therefore, must be evaluated carefully and thoughtfully before being acted on. Unfortunately, some of the data summoned in support of this claim are questionable: Studies claim that people must be sleep-deprived since most use alarm clocks to jolt themselves awake for resumption of their appointed tasks of the next day, rather than awakening naturally, out of satiation. The existence of the alarm clock as "proof" of sleep deficiency is like the early religious philosophers' argument for the existence of God: God must exist; otherwise, why would we have a name for Him . . . that is, "God!?" As additional evidence of chronic sleep deprivation, some have pointed to a significant subgroup of students who can sleep at any time if allowed to do so. But, as we discussed in Chapter 3, these kids normally nap, and late adolescents, subject to intense social interactive pressures, may indeed have some rather peculiar sleep patterns.

The point, as we have discussed earlier, is that there is a range of normal sleep patterns and that sleep needs vary. To quote Torriano: "Five hours sleep a traveller, seven a scholar, eight a merchant, and eleven every knave" (*Piazza Universale 114*. 1666). With documented sleep deprivation, lethargy, social withdrawal and irritability can set in after about 48 hours. But as we have also previously discussed, the issue that should be answered requires careful and controlled evaluation: How do personality type and temperament interact with sleep needs, and to what extent are abilities to cope and perform compromised by sleep loss? After 100 hours of sleep deprivation, under controlled conditions, reversible psychotic thinking, but little else, manifested itself in experimental subjects. Additionally, no residual impairment of brain function was seen once a 12-hour sleep-recovery period was undergone. These caveats notwithstanding, anxiety, rumination, tension, and preoccupation are psychological concomitants of the sleep deprivation accompanying chronic insomnia. Many sleep researchers, Anthony Kales and Joyce Kales among them, have suggested that particular personality characteristics lend themselves to the development of chronic insomnia in certain individuals. These folks, it is thought, tend to handle their emotional reactions to stressful situations by keeping them locked tight within (the euphemism "internalized" is a term that has been used to describe this behavior; it has been mistaken for an "explanation" rather than the "alternative rendering" that it really is). Such a response, it is thought, only keeps the outward dimensions of their reaction muted. Internally, the signs and symptoms of arousal and alarm persist, along with the disruption of sleep.

For any complaints of daytime sleepiness, one must consider the coexistence of other symptoms, such as fatigue, listlessness, morning headaches, night sweats, and changes in weight. For many medical and psychiatric conditions which present with low energy and fatigue, an important differential diagnostic clue is whether the complaint is really that of listless lethargy and fatigue or that of "hypersomnolence"—an excessive and prodigious sleepiness which comes on uncontrollably and in an untimely fashion, even while the individual is trying to stay awake. If the latter is present, and if other infectious, metabolic, psychiatric, and similar causes have been ruled out, one goes on to consider the disorders of excessive somnolence (DOES).

> It has been estimated that, of the more than 50,000 traffic fatalities that occur in the United States every year, as many as 15% may be caused by sleep-related disturbances. Sleep deprivation arising from shift work, circadian rhythm alterations, medical afflictions with and without use of medication, and drug and alcohol abuse can all lead to an increase in sleepiness and, when coupled with monotony and the lack of stimulus novelty or interest, can contribute to sleep-related automobile accidents. And the most common sleep-related causes of hypersomnolence are sleep apnea and narcolepsy.
>
> "Apnea" refers to the complete stoppage of airflow for more than 10 seconds at a time. There are three forms of sleep apnea. The first is "obstructive" apnea, the most common type, in which the individual continues to try to breathe, but an airway obstruction (from the nose down through the tonsils and below) leads to a decrease or cessation of airflow. Imagine recurrent episodes of airway blockage that lead to sudden, unanticipated disruptions in breathing every time you were just drifting off to sleep . . . maybe up to 50 times an hour or more! Even if you were not fully conscious of these multiple micro-awakenings after a while, you might certainly expect that the following day you would be pretty beat. The second form of apnea is called "central" apnea, and it involves the cessation of the respiratory effort itself (and, thereby, the flow of air). This is the most severe form of apnea, and Ondine's curse is one example. Here, the central nervous system controls of respiration are defective; there is no obstruction and with the consequent frequent awakenings, sufferers may complain of insomnia rather than of daytime hypersomnolence. The third variety of apnea is the "mixed" form, in which there is an initial failure in the endeavor to breathe followed by an obstruction of the upper airway.

COMPLAINTS OF EXCESSIVE SLEEPINESS AND OTHER DISORDERS OF REM SLEEP

Narcolepsy is a DOES which affects late teens and young adults primarily. However, it is also seen in a strain of beagle dogs, Labrador retrievers, poodles, Doberman pinschers, and even horses! The presence of the phenomenon in other species and the fact that it is seen in higher frequency among relatives of narcoleptics, suggest a strong biological, and perhaps genetic, basis for the disorder. In humans, the excessive daytime sleepiness of narcolepsy takes the form of sleep attacks: uncontrollable and unintended sleeping bouts, with immediate entry into REM sleep, lasting anywhere from 30 seconds to 20 minutes. There have been cases recorded where brief attacks such as these occur with a frequency of up to 200 a day! Some of these individuals may also experience episodes of automatic behavior, in which they can perform simple tasks and make plain, unadorned responses while maintaining complete amnesia for the period.

In addition to the sleep attacks and the extreme daytime sleepiness, many sufferers of narcolepsy also have a triad of symptoms including cataplexy, sleep paralysis, and hypnagogic hallucinations. Cataplexy is the sudden loss of muscle tone, occurring spontaneously or immediately following a strong emotional outburst. It affects the muscles responsible for maintaining posture so that after an energetic visceral eruption, the individual collapses like a marionette whose strings were cut, only to recover completely within a minute. Very recently (Siegel, 1991), a colony of cells, responsible for the onset of cataplexy in dogs, was discovered, distinct from, but in very close proximity to, the brainstem centers triggering REM sleep. Studies such as this one will lead us to further understand the interaction and communication among neurological command centers. Additionally, we will come to understand the important role of sequential timing of the activities of different centers in the orchestration of patterns of behavior.

Sleep paralysis can occur in normal individuals with no indication of narcolepsy. It is marked by the transitory presence of muscular paralysis. And hypnagogic hallucinations are vivid, dream-like images, occurring with the onset of sleep ("hypnopompic" is the name given to a similar phenomenon occurring upon awakening from sleep) and sometimes associated with anxiety. Again, this phenomenon can occur in people without the associated events that warrant a diagnosis of narcolepsy. Both hypnagogic and hypnopompic phenomena raise interesting questions about the nature of the experiences people have during different twilight states of arousal (whether induced by external agents in the peyote rituals of the desert Indian or the anesthesiologist's soporific elixir; whether caused by internal metabolic changes affecting cerebral nutrition and oxygenation, or evoked by willful cognitive exercises). Some suggest that many symptoms of narcolepsy, in particular, the narcoleptic triad, indicate a spill-over of REM sleep phenomena into waking life. One might further wonder whether certain dissociative states (with names such as depersonalization, fugue state, and multiple personality disorder), meditation trances, and ecstatic religious visions also represent split off cognitive fragments emerging from the REM state. Interestingly, both depression and narcolepsy involve a foreshortening of the REM latency period, indicating once again how nature's broad-spectrum phenomenon, called "depression," touches on a sleep disturbance.

As with sleep apnea, the narcoleptic individual suffers an irresistible urge to nap which suddenly overcomes him or her. But unlike sleep apneics, the narcoleptic usually awakens from the brief nap feeling refreshed. In addition to this response to a bout of daytime sleep, the presence or absence of the above-mentioned symptomatic triad, and the characteristic age of incidence, narcolepsy can be differentiated from the sleep apneas by the polysomnogram—the simultaneous monitoring of brain waves (EEG), eye movements (EOG, or electroculogram), and muscle tone (EMG, or electromyogram), with simultaneous recording of nasal airflow, oxygen levels in the blood, and respiratory-related movements of the chest and abdomen.

Two other conditions, which can cause hypersomnolence, involve movement disorders occurring during sleep. In the first, called, appropriately enough, periodic leg movements (PLM), irresistible movements of one or both legs take place during NREM sleep in a repetitive series of 30-second bursts, running consecutively for up to 45 minutes at a time. The other, called nocturnal myoclonus (for the spasmodic, jerky muscular contractions characteristic of it) also occurs during NREM sleep but is less well-understood than PLM. Both can be associated with DIMS or DOES, or with neither.

> The bone-chillingly eerie sound, like harsh gravel being pulverized, can jolt the sleeping partner awake. It is the sound of repetitive grinding, gnashing, clicking, and gritting of the teeth; it occurs in almost 10 percent of the adult population, and it is called bruxism (from the Greek, meaning, literally, to grind the teeth). These jaw

movements are purposeless (although they can have destructive dental consequences) and occur during the lighter stages of NREM sleep, although occasionally during REM sleep as well. The causes of bruxism are not known, but some feel that those individuals with chronically-aroused personalities—the so-called "Type A" personalities who may be assertive or retiring but who show a continuous aggressiveness, an ambition driven by underlying insecurity, and a time-pressured existence—are less able to cope flexibly with stressful situations and are somehow more susceptible to the nonfunctional expression of muscular tension during periods of decreased arousal wherein the degree of muscular disengagement is fluid and shifting.

A final word about muscular movements during sleep: it seems paradoxical but REM sleep, notable for the disengagement of muscle groups and the fall-off of muscle tone, is also characterized by the presence of ostensibly purposeless muscle twitches. This apparent inconsistency reflects the underlying paradoxical drama of REM sleep itself: the generalized activation of the brain, including just about every neurophysiological system assisting in motor activity but, at the same time, a simultaneous compensatory inhibition and blockage of the transmission of this "activation" so that the ultimate translation of the increased neuronal cellular activity into coordinated behavior is prevented. This disengaging "clutch" mechanism has been hypothesized to reside at the synaptic cleft, between connecting neuronal cells, and operates via mechanisms yet to be discovered. Investigators have suggested that the REM sleep twitches may be manifestations of this activated but disengaged process of REM sleep. As Chase and Morales, two researchers from the University of California at Los Angeles School of Medicine, said ". . . these concurrently active but diametrically opposed processes . . . could reflect . . . adaptive responses to a widely activated nervous system; it seems logical for the organism to protect itself from the deleterious consequence of undirected and inappropriate movements when it is blind and unconscious" (Chase and Morales, 1983).

Back in the late 60's it was reported that adults will "feed," if allowed unrestricted access to food or drink in an unstructured setting, every 90 minutes or so. Whether this suggestion will hold up to more rigorous examination of the possible rhythms of "free-running" eating behavior, remains to be seen. However, isolated reports, one of which was published by Scottish psychiatrist Ian Oswald (1986), presented the case of a man who, every 90 minutes, in synchrony with REM sleep, would briefly awaken, raid his refrigerator, and then drift back to sleep even as he was munching on the last remnants of his snack. This phenomenon may be part of a recently recognized large category of parasomniac disorders known as REM sleep behavior disorder (RBD). Like other manifestations of RBD, it involves complex motor activity (which appears somewhat purposeful) which occurs during REM sleep, when muscle tone is supposed to be reduced. The diagnostic criteria for RBD were first defined in the late 1980's and included the presence of behaviors which were out of line for sleep, accompanied by vivid dreams and a loss of the usual decrease in muscle tone expected during REM sleep. The disorder was present mostly in older males, and was frequently associated with some form of primary neurological disease.

So, a previously unrecognized group of disorders was discovered which involved a disruption in the normal **dis**connection which occurs between the brain activity and the muscular apparatus during REM sleep. The result is that the dreams seem to be acted out and the activity engendered seems to be purposefully directed by the dream thoughts. We do not know what the mechanism is underlying this peculiarity, nor do we yet know whether this deviance from usual sleep behavior, coupled with close observation of the dreams reported by the individual encountering this anomaly, will provide us with some clarification of the mind–body linkages between dream cognition and sleep state.

Behaviors which appear purposeful, but which occur without the individual's conscious awareness, are called automatisms. Although they can take place during either awake periods or during sleep, the characteristic of the state which seems to permit these behaviors to arise is the clouding of consciousness, with apparently consequent effects on awareness, established psychological inhibitions, and neurological restraints. A number of sleep-related disorders can be associated with such behaviors, and some of these behaviors can be violent. They have been reviewed in depth by Mahowald and coworkers (1990), and include sleepwalking, nighttime seizures, night terrors, RBD, sleep drunkenness, and some psychological conditions, perhaps following a traumatic event, and arising in relation to sleep. These last phenomena fall under the rubric of "dissociative states" (like the "multiple personality disorder," the amnesiac "fugue state," the focused attention of "trance," and the feelings of unreality associated with "depersonalization").

"Sleep drunkenness" seems to be one more example of the functional disconnection of sensory, cognitive, and muscle-effector systems that occurs during the transitions among the different stages of sleep and alertness. For instance, there is a difference in alertness between someone aroused directly from stage 3 or 4 sleep and someone else aroused from REM sleep: with the former, a state of confusion is often present initially; with the latter, the individual's reactivity to environmental stimuli is immediately right up to the speed of the normal waking state. This "confusional" state may have some relationship to sleep drunkenness, which refers to the presence of a transitory delerium-like quality to attention and cognition (usually associated with low levels of alertness), occurring while motor activity (usually associated with a high degree of alertness) persists. This disruption occurs during the change from sleep to waking, and can affect anyone. And whenever there is disorganized, unconstrained behavior, it is possible that some of it will have violent consequences. However, although it seems likely that violent behaviors can surface during episodes of "disconnected" states such as sleep drunkenness, it is not known whether these behaviors are goal-directed or can become so, or merely represent haphazard manifestations of a generally confused state without the benefit of its usual constraints. Even though as august an observer of the human condition as Plato stated, in *The Republic*, that "In all of us . . . there is a lawless, wild-beast nature . . ." that surfaces during sleep, that contention has not yet been substantiated in any way that would shed useful light on social and legal issues regarding responsibility and culpability for one's untoward acts.

AGING AND SLEEP DISORDERS

In view of the changes in the characteristics and quality of sleep that occur normally with aging, it is understandable, but problematic, for the elderly individual to look back and complain of sleep dissatisfaction based on a comparison to his or her earlier pattern. Just as with age-related changes in body-weight maintenance, or athletic prowess, or sexual endurance, the basis for the complaint is beyond appeal! Things ain't what they used to be! However, the existence of illness, situational factors, concurrent medications, and emotional disorders, in addition to disorders of sleep onset and maintenance and the parasomnias, can all interfere with sleep quantity and quality in different ways, at different epochs in an individual's life. For instance, sleep-disordered breathing is more prominent in older individuals, even those who are essentially physically well and have no evidence of sleep disruption. There are two natural developments in the sleep pattern as we age: (1) nighttime sleep normally becomes more fragmented and, depending on the extent of the fragmentation, daytime sleepiness may develop; and (2) our total nightly hourly sleep requirement decreases. Although women, on average, have more sleep complaints than men and are reported to use sleeping medication more than men, it is men who demonstrate, on close sleep lab observation, more changes in their sleep patterns with aging than women show. It would seem that what is operating here is a combination of gender-related physiological differences and of behavior deemed more permissible in one gender than the other.

Up to 50 percent of people over the age of 65 report some sleep-related difficulty, according to many different polls. In fact, sleep complaints are the second most common reason for an elderly person's doctor-visit (the first being symptoms related to an upper respiratory infection). From difficulty falling asleep, to difficulty staying asleep, and from breathing problems during sleep to early morning awakening, the frequency of complaints increases with the naturally evolving shift in sleep architecture. Just as there are age-related physical changes in body and organ functioning, so too there are naturally occurring age-connected changes in sleep and sleep-related phenomena. These may be based on changes in inherent sleep regulating centers found in the brainstem, on natural changes in the characteristics and regulation of circadian rhythms (an advance of the sleep phase creating a "night owl" pattern for some), and coupled with the concomitant appearance of medical or emotional disorders that may be more prevalent in later years. It is important to remember, however, that despite all the expected changes in the sleep cycle with age (including the change from biphasic sleep–wake cycle to the polyphasic sleep–wake–sleep–wake cycle), not all elderly people have subjective complaints of sleeplessness or disturbed sleep. And, in any case, insomnia is not a disease. It is a symptom, and a symptom that can represent many different underlying causes.

People over 65 years old are subject to much the same sleep-disruptive disorders that younger adults are, with several exceptions. One of these is the "sundown syndrome," mentioned briefly

earlier. The clinical picture is one of agitation and confusion at
sundown, with nighttime wandering and an increase in the incidence of the sleep apnea syndrome. Associated with the apnea
comes a sense of morning exhaustion, daytime sleepiness, confusion, and perhaps a transitory loss of muscular coordination,
headaches, a loss of sexual interest, and personality changes.

> Snoring, associated with sleep-related respiratory problems like
> apnea, can create marital problems. It is loud. It is disruptive. The
> noise, plus the irregular breathing pattern, can leave the awakened
> bed partner alert, listening for the next, irregular, and delayed
> inspiratory breath. And of course the residual daytime effects take
> their toll as well.
>
> Normal snoring in the healthy elderly individual is continuous
> and undulating in intensity. The snoring of the sleep apneic is
> extraordinarily loud, nonfluctuating in intensity, and discontinuous,
> with intermittent periods of breathing cessation lasting longer than
> 10 seconds each.

An additional factor in the production of sleep problems for
the elderly has been the use, and perhaps overuse, of sleeping
medications. In taking sleeping pills (and almost 40 percent of the
adult population have done so on a reasonably regular basis at
some time in their lives) the elderly can develop drug tolerance
and side effects (because of age-induced changes in body metabolism) and they can experience problems of drug interactions with
other medications taken.

A final word about a phenomenon that occurs after going to
bed but before going to sleep: a pins-and-needles-like uncomfort-
able sensation deep within the legs which is accompanied by an
urge to rub or move the legs vigorously to relieve the feeing. The
cause of this "restless leg syndrome" is not known, although it has
been seen in conjunction with diabetes, vitamin deficiencies,
chronic kidney disease, and circulatory problems of the legs. It is
different from, but may coexist with, nocturnal myoclonus, which
we spoke about earlier.

HEADACHES AND SLEEP

> Preceded by temporary visual disturbances from blinding flashes to
> descending curtains or blind spots, migraine attacks are severe
> throbbing headaches, often on one side of the head or over the eyes,

and accompanied frequently by nausea, and sensitivity to bright lights and loud noises. There are many variations on this symptomatic theme. Migraines can come on at any time and, in the susceptible individual, in response to triggers like stress, hunger, alcohol or chocolate consumption, or menstruation. They can be relieved by sleep, if they are daytime in origin; but some seem to be precipitated by sleep or relaxation. These headaches would be considered to be a "parasomnia"—an event not directly related to sleep-inducing or sleep-maintaining mechanisms, but occurring during sleep, or made worse by the interposition of sleep.

Coming in clusters of up to months at a time before subsiding, "cluster headaches" are one-sided, knife-like excruciating head pains affecting men more often than women, and can come on at the same time everyday. Like migraines, they can wake an individual out of a sound sleep.

One-third of the daytime cluster attacks begin during periods of relaxation, and a number of other headaches can arise regularly, in the early morning, perhaps as part of a syndrome associated with one or another of the parasomnias—offering intriguing hints regarding the relationship of headaches and pain perception to a basic rest–activity cycle, or BRAC. This cycle was initially proposed by Kleitman (1983) to be composed of brief (90-minute) but regularly recurring alterations in the level of activation of the central nervous system throughout the 24-hour day. This pattern would look, graphically, like an oscilloscope's S-shaped sine-wave, with peaks of activity and valleys of rest. And during sleep, the activation part of the cycle would be manifested as REM.

With regard to the putative interplay among headaches and a rest–activity cycle, let us then look again at our old friend, the neurotransmitter serotonin. We now note that not only is serotonin an important participant in neurochemical systems involved with sleep onset, mood regulation, and appetite adjustment, but it also plays an active role in modulating reactivity to painful stimulation. Decreased serotonin activity can be associated with increased difficulty in getting to sleep, depression, increased reactivity to painful stimuli, the narrowing of blood vessels, and perhaps, as suggested by Barabas and co-workers (1983), changes in the transitions among sleep stages (thereby accounting for some of the disruptions leading to the parasomnias).

Cluster headaches, if nocturnal, begin most often after a few hours of sleep have elapsed. Along with the excruciating pain can come a runny nose, tears, and pain in the eyeball itself. A number of different treatments have been tried, including the element lithium, used in its salt form previously to treat manic–depressive disorders, but here used in timed doses in an attempt to shift the chronology of circadian rhythms. Additionally, since sleep and relaxation have been observed to be factors present during the precipitation of these attacks, sleep deprivation has been tried as a treatment for cluster headaches. A variant of cluster headache, known as chronic paroxysmal hemicrania, characterized by a brief, but continuously recurring pain over one-half of the head, is responsive to another medication, indomethacin.

CHILDHOOD SLEEP PROBLEMS

Now I lay me down to sleep
I pray the Lord my soul to keep
And if I die before I wake
I pray the Lord my soul to take.

♦   ♦   ♦

By and large, children suffer the same primary sleep disorders that adults do, although with some differences related to developmental age. And in terms of the evolving patterns of sleep in the developing child, it is essential to remember that sleep in infants and preschool children is influenced by many environmental considerations, especially the behavior of parents. So why in the world would parents encourage a nighttime prayer, such as the one above, in a child?

To review for a moment an aspect of development which we touched on in Chapter 3: In the first year of life, particularly within the first 3 months, a "normal" infant will exhibit symptoms suggestive of gastrointestinal pain which occur periodically around the clock (not necessarily during sleep alone) but more commonly in the afternoon and evening hours. The baby will fuss and cry and awaken, if sleeping, with this "colic." Having outgrown this, the 1- to 3-year-old will still, "normally," have difficulty falling asleep. This time around, it is most likely due to an established psychological phenomenon known as separation anxiety. Here, because cognitive development has not yet permitted the child to maintain, over extended periods of time, conceptual representations and likenesses from the outside world, he or she has a fear of losing touch with that waking world and of being "separated from" the parent. This age marks the start of taking a favorite toy or blanket to bed, a "transitional object" from the outside world which helps to maintain a sense of continuity between the states of wakefulness and sleep. This is also the age of the start of bad dreams and nightmares (which reach a peak at 10–11 years of age). And in the young child with fears about going to sleep related to the separation anxiety, who then experiences a significant loss in his/her life and, as a result, begins to fuse as one, the preexisting confusion between sleep and death, this is the age when the seeds of a "death phobia" may be sown. It is not by accident that the bedtime prayer, quoted above, addresses the issue of death . . . the ultimate "separation" from life. Even the ancient Greeks acknowledged the primitive confusion of death with sleep . . . they considered the god of death, Thanatos, and the god of sleep, Hypnos, brothers!

Although these fears have been recognized to be almost universal at some point during early development, and their consequences for sleep (like difficulty falling asleep, frequent awakenings, nightmares, and talking in one's sleep) have likewise been appreciated, often, parental behavior, and in particular, inconsistent or inappropriate rituals established subtly around bedtime, reinforce the development of disrupted sleep patterns and an ability of the child to learn to soothe himself or herself to sleep. Traditionally it has been recommended that children do not sleep in the same bed with their parents. It has been said that such "co-sleeping" might foster "dependency," present untoward sexual stimulation, or provide an avenue for the expression of the parents' difficulties (with each other, with setting limits, or with their ambivalence about the responsibilities of parenting). With regard to this last point, let us not forget or underplay the significance of feelings stirred up by the temperamentally difficult child whose sleep pattern is indeed excessively disruptive for all concerned . . . a situation in which it may be unclear whether the sleep disturbance is a disturbance of the child or of the parent.

But, considering all these factors, it is important to note, first of all, that few cultures, other than western industrialized ones, expect their very young children to sleep by themselves, and, secondly, that co-sleeping in response to a child's sleep problem is different from co-sleeping because of living restrictions or cultural mores. There are no hard-and-fast rules regarding co-sleeping. The major guidelines consist of an awareness of the range of possible meanings of the behavior to both child and parent, and a sensitivity to the potential benefits and hazards of such an arrangement. So often, in situations such as this, expectations, more than anything else, determine whether certain practices become problems.

> The newborn infant needs time to develop the sleep architecture more characteristic of the adult pattern. It is not until the second year of life or so that the distinctive four stages of NREM sleep and REM sleep appear to establish themselves. Prior to that, infants show two rather amorphous periods co-mingled with periods of waking . . . "quiet" sleep and "active" sleep, forerunners of the NREM and REM stages to come.
>
> Back in 1981, Drs. Harper and Leake and their co-workers hypothesized that in these as yet fully formed infant sleep periods, there occurs a failure in an "arousal" mechanism such that, when respiratory difficulties arise for any one of a number of different possible reasons, the infant is unable to awaken sufficiently to correct its breathing problem, be it a mechanical obstruction or a precursor of an apneic disorder. Although intriguing as a hypothesis, the specific causes underlying the Sudden Infant Death Syndrome (SIDS) are not known. Estimates are that between five and ten thousand infants succumb to this syndrome each year in the United States (Thach, 1985; Lydic and Biebuyck, 1988).

Most sleep problems of childhood ultimately refer to anxieties about going to bed or to erratic habits developed around bedtime. But there are significant primary sleep disorders to be considered as well, and the most common of these in children fall under the category of the parasomnias. Whereas in adults, insomnia is the most common sleep complaint, in children bedwetting or enuresis (affecting 20–25 percent of all children), sleepwalking or somnambulism (occurring in approximately 3 percent of all youngsters), and night terrors or *pavor nocturnus* (the least common of the three) are the most prevalent complaints. All three parasomnias, along with sleep-talking (somniloquy), are NREM sleep phenomena, usually occurring only once a night, and usually during the first couple of hours of sleep, and decrease in frequency of occurrence with increasing age. This last observation has led many sleep specialists and pediatric neurologists to specu-late that these disorders represent developmental lags in the central nervous system, with the consequent errors in fine tuning being finally corrected when the normal maturational growth of neurons has been achieved by all the interlocking neurological systems.

Bedwetting is more common in boys and rarely continues into adulthood. The usual series of events occurs as follows: as the child is coming out of his first deep NREM sleep, and before entering his first REM stage, he exhibits some body movement, a slight increase in pulse rate and respiratory rate, and a penile erection. Then, 1–3 minutes later, during a relative calm, urina-tion occurs. Immediately following the urination, the child is typically difficult to awaken.

Sleepwalking occurs more in children (it is estimated that 2–3 percent of the adult population experiences bouts of somnambul-ism) and more in males. It can coexist with any of the other parasomnias or with the very rare, adult counterpart of night terror, called "incubus." The characteristic appearance of eyes open but glassy and "unseeing," as immortally portrayed by Shakespeare's Lady Macbeth, with clumsy movements and terse, mumbled communications, can last for several seconds or up to 30 minutes, and is usually accompanied by an amnesia for the event after the fact.

Night terrors present with a bloodcurdling scream in an inconsolable child who appears to be awake but cannot focus and is unresponsive to external intervention. They are relatively com-mon throughout the early school years and are, in fact, easier to handle than nightmares (although terrifying to witness) because, with night terrors, children are usually amnesiac and readily return to bed once the episode has subsided. With nightmares, the fears linger. The presence of confusion and subsequent amnesia are two additional points differentiating NREM sleep night ter-rors from REM sleep nightmares. Incidentally, both sleepwalking and night terrors can be precipitated in susceptible individuals . . . one by standing a child up during NREM sleep stage 3 or 4, the other by sounding off a loud noise during stage 3 or 4.

From this broad spectrum of sleep disorders, we have seen that the sleep mechanism is far from flawless. Furthermore, taking

into consideration all the different antecedents of sleep phenomena, we must keep in mind that the factors which may **cause** a
particular behavioral phenomenon (be it a disorder or not) are not
necessarily the same as those which then **maintain** its continuance.
The perturbations engendered by various vagaries and eccen-
tricities of the system were probably of little consequence to the
caveman who, like other mammals living relatively uncomplicated
(though perhaps perilous) lives of eating and resting, could make
up for minor disturbances by an additional postprandial nap. Not
so with modern-day work schedules, little league games, social
obligations, and commuting! Back then, a little additional sleepiness, while fishing or sitting by the fire, had nothing of the
potential consequences that being drowsy nowadays has, if that
drowsiness comes upon you while on a long and monotonous trip,
behind the wheel of an 8-cylinder gas-guzzler.

Chapter 10

Getting on a First-Name Basis with Mr. Sandman
Pills, Potions, and Remedies

A quiz: What do soothing hot showers, a warm glass of milk, the droning hum of the fan or air conditioner, and the well-worn Teddy Bear have in common? Answer: All are sleeping comforts, if not sleeplessness remedies, for selected individuals who may consider themselves to be "insomniacs." Another question: What distinguishes a mixture of white poppy seeds, lettuce seeds, balsam, saffron, and sugar, stewed in poppy juice, from modern-day recipes having fractured-dictionary names like Placidyl, Restoril, Compoz, or Halcion? The answer: about 500 years. The first is a formula proposed by Marsilio Ficino in his treatise *The Book of Life* written in 1489 (translated by Charles Baer) to remedy insomnia in intellectuals in whom "wasteful sleeplessness . . . leads to the drying out of their brains!" The latter are present-day pharmaceuticals which similarly promise relief and repose, and whose names inspire one to take Madison Avenue on with appelations for as-yet-to-be-developed pharmaceutical agents like: "Bon Appetit" . . . for the treatment of calcium-poor, postmenopausal women with osteoporosis; "Acro-Bat" . . . for combatting the fear and panic induced by high places; "Rectify" . . . for correcting constipation; or "Limber" . . . for use by the masseur as a cooling gel.

The search for elixirs of sleep moved, from the alchemist's workplace to the behavioral scientist's laboratory, when early electrophysiological studies first attempted to locate the centers in the brain that were presumed to control sleep. These studies progressed from electrical probings to surveys of energy utilization in these different areas, as techniques were devised that could peer into brain activity in a way analogous to that of the infra red-sensitive spy-in-the-sky satellites which locate hubs of activity below by detecting tell-tale signs of energy consumption. So, in the neuroscientist's laboratory, surveillance methods watched discrete areas of the brain for indications of changes in glucose consumption or protein synthesis during the transitions into and out of sleep. Interest had turned toward the underlying chemistry of the brain.

It was then just a matter of time before attention turned to the spectrum of behaviorally active chemical substances, classified as hypnotic and/or sedative because of their sleep-inducing properties. With these agents, attempts could be made to understand the regulation of the sleep cycle by directly introducing them into areas of the brain suspected to be important regulatory sites, and by using these chemicals as pharmacologic intermediaries or "tools," probing the functional patterns regulating different behavioral states.

So, interest in "sleeping pills" soared not just because of the pervasiveness of sleep concerns but also because these agents provided a further level of sophistication in the investigation of the phenomenon of sleep. In the course of such empirical investigation, it was discovered that the factors that trigger sleep onset may not be the same factors that support its maintenance, once it has begun. Additionally, as such explorations proceeded, receptor sites (or "locks") were found to exist in certain areas of the brain which were specifically responsive to man-made chemical "keys," known as benzodiazepines (two examples of which are more familiarly known by their brand names, Valium® and Librium®). Why, you might ask, would nature, early on in evolutionary time, create neurological mechanisms specifically responsive to drugs manufactured by pharmaceutical companies millenia later?

Well, of course, this turns out not to be a conspiratorial manifestation of a natural–industrial complex, analogous to

Eisenhower's renowned "military–industrial complex." Instead, a modern-day fabricated substance gets to the age-old receptor area on the surface of brain nerve cells and, because of structural similarities, is able to imitate the effect of naturally occurring substances, whose presence had been unsuspected until their aforementioned man-made cousins' action was discovered. These "benzodiazepine receptors," throughout specific areas of the nervous system, have been found to mediate important functions having to do with anticonvulsant activity, muscle relaxation, anti-anxiety effects, and the onset and maintenance of sleep.

Following from the initial bevy of neurochemical inquiries, it became clear that the array of sleep-related drug effects is broad. The intricate interweaving and cross-connecting of these effects is just beginning to be mapped onto a larger schematic representation of the neurochemistry of the brain. So before going on to talk of specific therapeutic agents and how they might be used, we should, just briefly, survey a spectrum of the current chemical agents of choice in dealing with a number of sleep-related problems. Benzodiazepines affect a neurotransmitter by the name of gamma aminobutyric acid (GABA), which in turn may influence and modulate the metabolic activity of serotonin. Hormones, such as progesterone and hydrocortisone, have effects on sleep which oppose each other. Medications used to treat depression initially decrease REM sleep but, with continued use, may result in an increase in both REM sleep and in stage 4 NREM sleep. Agents known as calcium channel-blockers prevent the sedative effects of the benzodiazepines. The secretion of growth hormone (GH) surges during the onset of sleep. Furthermore, some researchers have hypothesized the existence of some humoral factor or factors, some elixir of Morpheus, that forms or form the chemical basis for the regulation of sleep, both its onset and its maintenance.

Actually, the search first began in the early 1900's, when French physiologists deprived animals of sleep and then attempted to detect the presence of a sleep-inducing substance, produced by the brain in response to this deprivation, which might spill over into the bloodstream. An early experiment reported that it was possible to induce sleep in one animal by the transfusion of blood from its sleeping littermate. The conclusion was reached that a "sleep hormone" had been found in the blood that causes sleep to occur. Further experiments called cross-perfusion and cross-circulation studies followed. Borbely and To-bler (1989) report on one such experiment which, in initial description, is worthy of a Stephen King novel, but in findings clarifies the significance of sleep-inducing factors in the blood: A dog had a second head implanted so that the animal's circulatory system supplied blood to both heads; although such an experimental situation is not one that survives for more than several days, it was conclusively demonstrated that each head slept and woke independently of each other. The same was subsequently found to hold in an experiment of nature: human twins, joined at the head and sharing the same arterial blood supply, had totally independent sleep—waking cycles with no synchrony between them whatsoever.

The above results notwithstanding, continued search for humoral agents critical in the medication of the sleep—wake cycle has resulted in claims that the following substances may play a role in the regulation of sleep: prostaglandin, muramyl dipeptide (MDP), delta sleep-inducing peptide (DSIP), uridine, insulin, sleep-promoting substance (SPS), Factor S, vasoactive intestinal peptide (VIP), cholecystokinin octapeptide (CCK-8), growth hormone (GH), melatonin, serotonin, and acetylcholine. As can be seen by the makeshift nature of a number of these names, neither the chemical identity of some of these compounds nor their specific range of action has been completely uncovered as yet. When administered to humans with the purpose of promoting sleep, many of these compounds give results that are contradictory to those found in animal studies. And as an interesting side-note, some of these agents have specific but as yet inconsistently characterized effects on sleep, and well-substantiated effects on components of the body's immune-response system.

As we are talking about the role of humoral factors whose roles as sleep-promoting substances remain to be clarified, we should make it clear that these compounds fall into different categories. On the one hand we have neurotransmitters, like GABA, serotonin and acetylcholine. On the other hand we have hormones such as progesterone, growth hormone, and insulin. All are chemical compounds, operating at sites some distance in the body from where they were secreted. The former have direct actions on nerve cells, being specifically involved in the transmission of nerve signals across the synaptic cleft between cells. The latter coordinate larger functions by evoking responses in glands or organs, at distances from their point of secretion considerably larger than the microscopic ones of their neurotransmitter cousins. All the compounds discussed here represent naturally occurring, or endogenous, substances that mediate physiological operations and proceedings and, therefore, for the sake of our discussion here, are considered together as "humoral" agents.

While the neurochemists have raised new questions and presented new challenges to all researchers to tease apart and identify the complicated intertwined threads that hold together the story of sleep, they have also provided physicians with new and improved pharmacologic tools to add to their therapeutic armamentarium addressing sleep-related problems. And as advances made on the neurochemical front are being translated into clinically applicable information, increasing sophistication is slowly being added to physicians' prescription practices with regard to hypnotic medications.

THE SLEEPING PILLS

First prescribed, on a large-scale basis, were drugs with names like meprobamate (Miltown®) and the barbiturates (like Seconal® and Nembutal®), ethchlorvynol (Placidyl®), glutethimide (Doriden®), methaqualone (Quaalude®), and methyprylon (Noludar®), all of which, although different in chemical structure, were capable of producing the following: addiction and paradoxical excitement (particularly in the elderly), a "rebound" worsening of the sleep disturbance and danger of seizures upon discontinuance, and a serious lethal threat if taken in overdosage! In addition, some of these agents were capable of creating serious and detrimental interactions with other drugs the patient might have been taking. But they did promote sleep in some form. For a presumed safer alternative, physicians often resorted to either chloral hydrate (the hypnotic ingredient in "knock-out drops" or a "Mickey Finn") or the antihistamines (like Benadryl® or Vistaril®). The latter compounds, still used by some as soporifics, are only mildly sedating, being much less effective than currently available hypnotic drugs. Additionally, they carry with them the possibility of substantial side-effects.

Then came the benzodiazepines, and with them the possibility of a refined appreciation of the indications and contraindications for specific hypnotic medications in specific clinical circumstances. The different species within this chemical group differ in terms of what is called their pharmacokinetics, how fast they get absorbed into the body once they are ingested, and then how quickly they get to the sites of action and become engaged before they are broken down by various metabolic processes into inert component by-products.

With regard to the benzodiazepine family of compounds, there are essentially three categories of substances distinguished by how quickly they reach peak blood levels after being taken: the longer-acting (like flurazepam or Dalmane®) achieves maximum blood levels in 90 minutes or less, but the effects of one dose remain active in the body for several days (so that with repeated use, a net accumulation of drug effect may lead to a spillover into daytime sleepiness); the intermediate-acting (like temazepam or Restoril®) with a slower onset of action, reaches peak blood levels in 2–3 hours, and its effects are eliminated from the body within a day's time, but it may be less effective (because of its slower absorption) for treating someone who has difficulty getting to sleep; and the short-acting variety (like triazolam or Halcion®), which has a relatively rapid onset as well as a very short duration of action and, as such, can possibly run its course before awakening time, thereby resulting in early morning, rebound insomnia.

These medications, although much more benign than the older categories of hypnotic medications, are not without potentially confounding side-effects. And it is up to the experienced clinician to assess the indications for, and the efficacy of, each particular hypnotic agent, taking into account the possibility of daytime drowsiness leftover from the previous night's dosage, the abuse potential of the drug, the side-effect profile of the particular agent, and the medical condition of the individual that might provide contraindications for the particular drug's use. Monitoring daytime functioning is an essential part of the clinical process involved in evaluating sleep medications. Unfortunately, it is still not uncommon today to hear of a patient with a 1- or 2-year history of sleep difficulties who, after several abortive attempts at self-treatment (confining himself to bed, engaging in vigorous exercise before bedtime to "exhaust" himself, trying various over-the-counter remedies, and eventually engaging in daytime napping "to take the edge off the discomfort"), gets himself to a doctor who prescribes a hypnotic drug, which at first seems to help, but quickly loses its effect. With increasing discomfort and anxiety, the patient escalates his insistence for more medication, and eventually receives increasing doses or the addition of a new hypnotic agent, with the story repeating its destructive spiral downward toward drug dependence while the presenting symptomatology remains unchanged or worsens.

We are becoming more knowledgeable about the processes affecting the sleep–wake cycle and are becoming more sophisticated in our approach to the evaluation and treatment of the disruptions in this cycle. But we are "becoming" . . . we are not "there" yet, so research continues to attempt to delineate particular indications for specific hypnotic drug use. A general summary of our current state of knowledge supports the following indications:

1. For normal sleepers who experience a brief, transitory episode of difficulty sleeping in response to a clearly identifiable precipitant (jet lag, presurgery jitters, or stage fright)—either tolerate the disruption with no medication or give a very limited course of a short-acting benzodiazepine (like triazolam).

2. For a brief period of insomnia (like (1) above, also related to an external event or loss and also involving difficulty falling asleep and/or staying asleep, but lasting somewhat longer)—evaluate and correct "sleep hygiene" (see below), coupled perhaps with a brief course of hypnotic medication, taken intermittently and stopped after two nights of "satisfactory" sleep.

3. For the individual who either misperceives his sleep need or who has displaced onto the sleep process a reaction of anxiety and arousal that had been previously associated with a traumatic event, and who therefore suffers from a chronic disruption in his sleep pattern, sometimes called "conditioned insomnia" (like Pavlov's dog, mentioned in the previous chapter, which salivated when he heard the bell ring, our sleep sufferer, here, responds to

the stimulus of the bedtime setting with apprehension and awakening)—evaluate and correct "sleep hygiene" and bring to bear the range of behavioral interventions (see below). Do **not** use currently available hypnotic agents.

4. With night terrors, sleepwalking and sleep talking in children—since benzodiazepines alter the configuration of sleep architecture (namely, they suppress stage 4 NREM sleep and REM sleep), they have been used with these disorders. So too have certain antidepressant medications (which also have been used in treating bedwetting, and seem to have effects on some aspects of sleep similar to that of the benzodiazepines). If an adult presents with these symptoms, a psychiatric evaluation is always indicated.

5. With insomnia associated with severe medical conditions, one must (as always) search for the underlying factors responsible for the sleep disturbance. These factors can be diverse, and the solution to the sleep problem resulting from them depends on a specific identification of the individual phenomenon. Consider a devastating physical illness like cancer, for example. Whether one is up all night because of pain, is unable to sleep because of the nausea or specific central nervous system toxic effects induced by various chemotherapeutic agents, or whether one is suffering from the direct effects of a cancer or the indirect psychological and social effects of being ill—all can trigger disturbed behavior and sleep patterns which can be addressed therapeutically once the underlying cause has been clearly identified. Some have reported that aspirin effectively alleviates minor sleep complaints, on a short-term basis. Whether this is so, and, if it is so, what the mechanism might be by which such an effect is achieved (whether it is related to effects on body temperature patterns or the freeing up of stores of tryptophan, the amino acid precursor of serotonin that we spoke of in Chapter 6) remains to be determined. However, an interesting additional claim, that the discontinuance of aspirin after a 2-week period of constant use may result in a "withdrawal insomnia," underscores the importance of carefully evaluating people with a complaint of insomnia who may have been receiving regular doses of aspirin for heart disease or arthritic conditions.

6. The treatment of narcolepsy involves the use of both pharmacological and nonpharmacological approaches: Whereas

stimulant drugs are used by some, and both tricyclic antidepressant medications (like imipramine or Tofranil®) and an agent called gamma-hydroxybutyrate have been used to suppress the REM portion of sleep, nondrug treatment of the possible precipitant conditions (including the psychological states of over-excitability or boredom in response to conditions of stress or monotony) is a crucial aspect of the therapeutic regimen.

7. In most people who have conditions of unusual muscle or motor behavior during sleep, these conditions are not attributable to psychiatric disease. Periodic leg movements (PLM) and REM behavior disorder (RBD), parasomnias discussed in Chapter 9, are treated with the drug clonazepam (Klonopin®) but, on clinical grounds alone, these conditions are sometimes difficult to distinguish from nocturnal seizures or even bouts of sleep terror or sleepwalking (for which the treatment would be different). Therefore, careful pretreatment evaluation is emphasized.

8. And finally, for those with depression-related disorders, some other drugs are used primarily but not exclusively in treatment and, therefore, have secondary effects on sleep. There is a full range of antidepressant medications, and some that are not classically considered such (like valproate and ethyl alcohol . . . the latter being a depressant in its own right and the most commonly used nonprescription sleep "medication." It has little curative ability and much addictive power and, as such, its prolonged or habitual use represents a potential disaster, and disease itself, just waiting to happen).

THE TREATMENT OF INSOMNIA

With regard to "insomnia," Hippocrates recognized four centuries B.C., that it ("agrypnia") resulted from suffering and the throes of life. He considered it also to be a normal concomitant of the aging process. But the subjective and anecdotal report of "poor sleep" is notoriously inaccurate at worst and unclear at best. For instance, when comparing subjective reports about sleep with objective measures, the following discrepancy obtains: the subjective complaints of insomnia in four out of five individuals cannot be confirmed by current measures available in the sleep lab.

According to Carskadon and co-workers (1976), most people observed in the sleep lab who have such complaints sleep about 30 minutes longer than they estimate and fall asleep 30 minutes more quickly than they think they do. In addition, Carskadon noted that normal individuals, whose nightly sleep time is reduced to a maximum of 5½ hours even for long periods of time, do not show any marked effect on performance or mood.

The point is that insomnia is a common symptom and it is multidetermined in all ages, both in terms of who suffers from it and when that particular individual chooses to voice the complaint. It is found in both the weak and the strong, the normal as well as the abnormal. It is not in and of itself a "disease." Rather it is a symptomatic complaint used to describe a condition, or perception, of sleep defect or deficiency. This reflection of change in underlying physiological regulation or psychological process may have many different possible causes, ranging from environmental disruptions, to anxiety and physical illness; from depression and drug abuse, to the unsuspected side-effects of medications prescribed for other conditions; and from benign anticipatory excitement to an integral component of the normal aging process itself.

Sleep "problems" are common, and these complaints have led to a widespread search by many present-day Ponce de Leons, not for the fabled "fountain of youth," but instead for the elixir of sleep . . . what Iago called "the drowsy syrups" in his threat to Othello, and what current researchers and advertisers suggest might be called by the names we have briefly reviewed above. As such, over 200 million drugstore prescriptions were written for hypnotic medications over a 5-year period 15 years ago, according to a U.S. Department of Health survey. And the numbers have increased since then. More than one-half of the approximately 35 million patients who are admitted to general hospitals each year are given sleeping medication. Sleeping pills are, in fact, the most highly prescribed medication in the U.S. today.

Hypnotic drugs are indeed important therapeutic tools if employed wisely. On the one hand, there is a role for their brief, adjunctive use in symptomatic relief, but never in place of addressing the underlying causes of the sleep-related problem. The potential consequences of prolonged and careless use of these agents, on the other hand, are too costly. And what are some of these possible risks of their long-term usage (other than the increasing ineffectiveness, drug dependency, and the attendant diversion from dealing with factors underlying the complaint of insomnia)? Well, the following: untoward interactions with other medications, rebound insomnia with daytime anxiety, paradoxical agitation, respiratory suppression (a particular hazard in people with sleep apnea), memory impairment, withdrawal syndromes, confusion in the elderly (with falls and fractures possible), over-dosage in depression, compounding of a toxic state if the insomnia is caused by some organic agent or intoxicant, and the lowering of the ability to be aroused during times of crisis or alarm (like the smell of smoke, the cry of an infant, or the ring of the telephone). With this information as a caution, it is still important to recognize that hypnotic medications are powerful tools that provide an important therapeutic resource when it comes to sleep-related disorders.

In the treatment of disorders of the sleep–waking cycle, the more resources one has, the wider the range of therapeutic choices one is afforded. The purpose of this chapter is not to make junior doctors out of us all, nor to encompass the enormous complexity of interlocking phenomena and translate the complex interwoven information, from all the different disciplines that impinge on the issues surrounding disorders of the sleep–wake cycle, into bite-size and oversimplified tidbits that fall under the rubric of "self-help." The purpose, rather, is to render meaningful as much of the factual information that has been recently established about sleep and, as was suggested in Chapter 1, to demonstrate that control over one's own sleep and health is best achieved by becoming an enlightened "assistant diagnostician," aware of and open to the wealth of information available. Neither this chapter, nor the book in general, are to be taken as a close-cycle "how-to" tract purporting to offer the last word and ultimate authority on self-help.

As we have discussed earlier, all treatment begins with diagnosis. Only by careful description can we hope to match symptoms, and their underlying diseases and syndromes, to effective therapies. The key to most psychiatric diagnosis comes from the patient's history and the clinical interview with the individual. The same is true with sleep-disorder diagnosis. Essential in this data-gathering process is a careful and complete review of the medical and psychiatric record, in addition to the current clinical review. It is often helpful to have the patient keep a diary of sleep-related activities in preparation for further diagnostic evaluation. As an aid in organizing such a diary, and as a preliminary screening, I have patients fill out the following form, which I then review with them in depth:

ADULT SLEEP STATUS QUESTIONNAIRE (ASSQ)

Age _____ Sex _____ Weight _____ Marital status _____

Current occupation (including hours and degree of travel):

Occupational history, over past 10 years:

General health status, circle one: Excellent Good Fair Poor

Are you under a doctor's care for any condition?
    Please specify if "yes":

Frequency of visits to health-care professionals over past two
    years (List names and specialties):

Do you have any current health concerns?
    Please specify if "yes":

Any known allergies/sensitivities? _____
Are you taking any pills/supplements/medications, pre-
    scribed or not?
    Please specify if "yes":

Over the past 6 months, have you experienced any change in:
appetite/weight? _____
activities/interest? _____
significant relationships/concerns? _____
sexual interests/activity? _____

Would you consider yourself more a "cool/calm" person or an "energetic/high-strung" one? _____

Are you a worrier? _____ A go-getter? _____

Are you often impatient with yourself or others? _____
Do you feel a sense of time pressure? _____
Please explain:

Do you have frequent or noticeable shifts or changes in your mood? _____
Do you have a high-point and a low-point most days? _____
Please explain:

Describe type, frequency, and timing of any physical exercise:

How satisfied are you with your sleep? _____

Please note the following:
Usual bedtime on weekdays _____ On weekends _____
Usual arising time on weekdays _____ On weekends _____
Usual number of minutes taken to fall asleep on weekdays _____ On weekends _____

Does sleepiness or fatigue intrude into your daytime activity? _____
In any particular or recurrent pattern? _____
Please describe:

Describe what measures you have taken to deal with it:

Where you do sleep best? At home _____ Away from home _____

Describe the room in which you usually sleep with regard to noise, light, temperature, etc.:

Describe your pillow and mattress:

Do you sleep alone or with someone? _____ In the same bed? _____

Has your partner observed that you:
Breathe erratically or snore loudly? _____
Walk or talk in your sleep? _____
Seem disoriented or confused entering/exiting sleep?
_____
Are unduly restless in your sleep? _____

Does you partner have a sleeping problem? _____ If "yes", explain:

Describe your bedtime routine:

Has your sleep pattern changed recently? _____
Please specify in what way:

Do you nap? _____ Regularly? _____ What time of the day? _____ When during the week? _____
How long are your naps? _____

How soon before bed do you eat something? _____

Do you have difficulty staying awake during the day? _____
    Please explain:

Do you have difficulty getting to sleep? _____

Do you have difficulty staying asleep through the night?
_____
    Please describe the frequency and length of these epi-
    sodes, and whether they are associated with any other
    symptoms or problems:

Do daytime worries keep you up at night? _____
    What sort?

Are you able to sleep as an "escape" from worry? _____

Do you snore? _____

Do you have recurrent dreams with the same theme? _____
    If yes, please describe:

Do you have disturbing dreams frequently? _____

Do you have heartburn? _____ Palpitations? _____
    Muscle/joint pains? _____ Leg twitches? _____
    Difficulty breathing? _____ Urinary urgency?
    _____ Hunger pangs? _____ Night sweats?
    _____ Jaw/dental problems? _____

Do you take anything to help you sleep now? _____
Do you smoke? _____ How much and when:

How much alcohol do you drink, and when:

Do you consistently awaken very early in the morning?
_____

Describe what you do if you cannot sleep (including both thoughts and activities):

To what do you attribute your sleeping difficulty?

What remedies have you tried in the past? (Please note how successful they were and for what period of time):

Is there a history of sleep problems in your family? _____
Insomnia? _____ Bedwetting? _____ Sleep-walking/talking? _____ Narcolepsy? _____
Depression? _____

The importance of information gleaned from such questions, and followed up by a direct one-on-one interview, cannot be emphasized enough in terms of the healing process itself and with regard to the evaluation and practical care of sleep problems. The strategies that most people come up with to attempt to remedy a bout of sleeplessness (like spending more time in bed or taking daytime naps and drinking lots of coffee to get through the day) are self-defeating, to put it mildly. Some are just mildly amusing in their idiosyncrasy: Charles Dickens reportedly always made sure that his bed ran parallel to a north–south axis in an 1800-rendition of the belief that beneficial effects were to be reaped from the proper alignment with the earth's magnetic forces. More recently, Winston Churchill is said to have slept, when possible, with a spare bed in his room for use if his bed linens became too disheveled or warm for his sleeping comfort.

Nonetheless, it remains axiomatic that knowledge and the careful delineation of the problem through self-appraisal are the first steps toward improvement. To understand anyone's sleep complaint, it is essential to understand the larger context of his/her daily life. The more specialized tools included in polysomnography (the electroencephalograph, the electro-oculograph, the electromyograph, the electrocardiograph, and techniques for the measurement of respiration, blood levels of oxygen, and electrical skin conductance), as well as specialized medical tests (including holter monitoring of heart function throughout a 24-hour period and procedures to evaluate penile erection capability), multiple sleep latency tests, and specialized neuropsychological evaluations, and the audiovisual recording of behaviors . . . all ultimately available, through the sleep specialist, to the sufferer of a sleep-related problem, must await the initial, and **essential**, clinical evaluation. So, if you are concerned about some aspect of your sleep, hone your observational skills and organize what you see by going through the ASSQ. Then, in the context of what you have already read, you can better and more knowledgeably consider your next step in consultation with an authority on sleep disorders.

Incidentally, the same is true for the evaluation of suspected sleep-related disorders in children. However, with both the evaluation and subsequent treatment of sleeping problems in children, the parents' participation must be enlisted. To aid in this, the sleep status questionnaire has been adapted for children, to be filled out by parents:

CHILD SLEEP STATUS QUESTIONNAIRE (CSSQ)

Age _____ Sex _____ Weight _____ Height _____
Grade level _____

Nickname/special family name: _____
Sibling order and ages:

School history (if relevant):

General health status, circle one: Excellent Good Fair Poor

Is this child under a doctor's care for any condition? _____
   What has been the frequency of visits to health-care professionals over the past 6–12 months? _____
   Explain:

Is this child currently taking any pills or medications/ supplements, whether prescribed or not? _____ Any allergies? _____ Please specify:

Family history: Is anyone under a doctor's care for any condition? _____
Is there a family history of sleep problems? (Consider insomnia, bedwetting, depression, narcolepsy, sleep-walking, sleep talking):

Are there current family stresses, conflicts or adversities? (Consider health-related, interpersonal, job/financially-related, etc.):

With regard to this child:
How do his/her growth and development compare with older and younger siblings?:

How do his/her personality and temperament compare with parents', siblings', and other children's or peers'?:

How would you describe this child's temperament, personality and energy level?:

How would you describe your own?:

Any recent changes in this child's interests, activity level, appetite or interactions? _____
List parental concerns about this child's health or behavior, if any:

Parental concerns about child's sleep:
    Mother's:

    Father's:

Describe bedroom (bed, roommates, noise, temperature, light):

Describe napping patterns (frequency, timing and length):

How does the family deal with bedtime? Describe routines:

Please note child's sleep-related behavior, as follows:
    Usual bedtime: Consistent?_____
    Usual arising time: Consistent?_____
    Specific nighttime routines:

    Observed behavior at bedtime (including protestations, self-soothing, specific fears voiced, thumbsucking, head-rocking/banging):

    Observed nighttime behaviors (like muscle jerks, teeth grinding, anxiety attacks or terrors, walking, talking, bedwetting):

    Observed daytime sleepiness:

How often does the child sleep in the same bed as parent(s)?
_____ Describe typical occasion:

What remedies have been tried in the past? Please describe
how successful they were, and for how long:

So we have now embarked on a course of evaluation with the ultimate goal to achieve the therapeutic alleviation of a sleep-related disorder. Let's begin with the complaint of insufficient sleep. And for the sake of discussion, let us define insomnia by some concrete, practical criteria, mindful of the fact that these criteria are not hard and fast and that there is much variation among individuals both in terms of what might constitute sleep loss and what might comprise sufficient discomfort to warrant a complaint of sleep loss. Let us consider "insomnia" to be present if any one of the three following criteria is approximated: an individual takes more than one hour to fall asleep, each night's sleep is interrupted more than two or three times and is accompanied by difficulty in returning to sleep, and/or the individual sleeps no more than 3 or 4 hours a night.

We all reflect on the sufficiency of our sleep, and many of us feel that our sleep is inadequate. But not all of us who feel that way consider ourselves insomniacs. Certainly some 40 hours of continuous sleep deprivation can be tolerated by most of us with little or no residual consequence once sleep has been reinstituted. In fact, it is not until at least twice that amount of continuous deprivation has occurred that significant behavioral disturbances can become apparent. These too, however, are rapidly reversible with the reintroduction of sleep.

THE EFFECTS OF SLEEP DISRUPTION

The aforementioned notwithstanding, there are consequences to sleep disruption (as we reviewed in Chapters 4 and 5) and it may be that the fragmentation of the sleep cycle is more important in determining these consequences than the absolute amount of sleep actually gotten or lost. For instance, one night's sleep loss results in a decreased ability to deal with novel situations in a flexible and creative way. At times of sleep deprivation, we apparently tend to fall back on more rigid, preestablished patterns of response. This has been assumed to be a reflection of a loss in "creative ability." In fact what it may present us with, incidentally, is an opportunity to understand a little more about what the components of "creativity" might be. What seems to suffer as a result of sleep deprivation is spontaneity in dealing with new, strange, or novel situations. What has been called "convergent thinking"—the ability to deal with familiar tasks which require nothing more than the implementation of familiar, previously proven behaviors— remains unaffected. A sleep-deprived rural mechanic may not be able to solve a gas-line problem in a new-fangled fuel-injected sedan, but he can quite easily service a familiar carburetor in an older model car. But "divergent thinking," the spontaneous, free-wheeling quality characteristic of creative thinking, does suffer from sleep disruption, and this loss is not compensated for by the inherent interest in the task or by applying increased motivation to perform from without. Its loss appears to be corrected only by the replenishment of sleep.

As has already been mentioned, the key to improving the sleep of insomniacs is diagnostic evaluation or assessment . . . considering the entire range of possible medical, psychological, and situational or environmental factors that may contribute to the onset or maintenance and perpetuation of a sleep disturbance. Insomnia is a common phenomenon which is multiply determined and presents with varying clinical pictures of severity and duration. But one doesn't just treat the complaint of insomnia, or of daytime sleepiness either for that matter.

Since there are many different causes of insomnia, as well as many different conditions determining the circumstances under which an individual will actually make his/her complaint of sleeplessness known, no one treatment suffices. A clear description of the problem must be obtained from both the patient and his/her partner. Any relevant psychological factors must be evaluated, including what the patient expects with regard to his/her sleep. Then a treatment approach incorporating, most likely, a number of different therapeutic interventions will stand a better chance of providing a satisfactory clinical outcome.

The menu from which such interventions are selected is broad: from the improvement of habitual behaviors surrounding sleep (called, quaintly enough, "sleep hygiene") via education, counseling or psychotherapy, to the institution of behavioral methods (with names such as stimulus control, relaxation training, paradoxical intention, guided imagery, self-instruction, token reinforcement, and biofeedback); from the use of "electrosleep," low-energy radio emission therapy, or "sleep restriction," to the use of hypnosis and the manipulation of exposure to environmental light; from the adjunctive use of dietary components, teas, and tonics, to the employ of modern hypnotic medications . . . the therapeutic modalities available to the clinician are numerous, and effective, if judiciously applied.

IMPORTANT ISSUES IN TREATMENT

Oftentimes the initial task in both the diagnosis and treatment of insomnia is to overcome the insomniac's denial of the presence of psychological issues underlying the sleep problem. Of course there are primary sleep disturbances with a basic biological foundation, but it is by now well-established that psychological elements (what some might prefer to call "emotional conflicts") are fundamental to many forms of adult sleep disorders. With children, sleep disorders may have developmental in addition to environmental and parental factors at their core. With adults, the psychological often plays a larger role.

Take for example the elderly individual in whom we have come to expect certain "normal" changes in the sleep cycle. Although decreased sleep satisfaction, the phase advance of sleep, the loss of stages 3 and 4 of NREM sleep, increased daytime sleepiness, and the presence (perhaps in mild or subclinical form) of primary sleep disorders, all are concomitants of increasing age, one should not automatically assume that "aging" explains all complaints of insomnia in the elderly. In fact, the complaint of insomnia may not be the consequence of physiology at all, but rather of responses to environmental factors . . . like a constricted daily routine with no outside interests, isolation in a deteriorating neighborhood, or perhaps living with a chronically-ill spouse who demands constant care. The whole range and spectrum of daily living conditions impact on a person's life. It is hardly surprising then that all aspects of life might be affected, including the one-third of which we spend in, or near, sleep.

Before turning to a review of the "nondrug" approaches to the treatment of sleep disorders, let us just reexamine three issues regarding the use of medications. First of all, it should be remembered that "sleeping pills" (except in certain primary dyssomnias) are nonspecific reducers of symptoms. However, even though they may offer only symptomatic relief and may not treat the underlying disorder, in certain situations a brief and careful prescription of medication, used in conjunction with other treatment interventions, can be useful. Cases in point include acute trauma, the sleep disruption accompanying myoclonic leg jerks and, at times, early stages of a jet lag syndrome.

Secondly, relying on pills alone to "reduce stress," for example, and thereby to enhance sleep, can backfire. There is no pill to "cure" the problems of living. Medication can help in the modulation of physiological responses to stressful challenges, but it does not get rid of stress. Stress is a part of life and a welcome part at that. It forms the challenge from which we grow and become better problem-solvers. The therapeutic emphasis with "stress" must be to reduce **distress** by living through, and coping with, stress.

Thirdly, in usual sleep laboratory studies, the effectiveness of hypnotic drugs is far from spectacular. Gillin and Byerly (1990, see reference for chapter 9) summarized the findings: total sleep time increases by only 30 minutes during the first three nights of treatment. Now, as has been mentioned, total sleep time (as compared with sleep fragmentation and variability from night to night) may not be the critical point differentiating between a person's satisfaction with his sleep and calling himself an insomniac. So whether an individual is a Thomas Edison, George Bernard Shaw, Napoleon, or a Darwin-like night owl on the one hand, or an Einstein-like slug-a-bed on the other, is probably less important than the quality of the actual time spent sleeping. To what extent various hypnotic agents can differentially affect the composition of the sleep cycle in a therapeutic fashion remains to be determined. It just must be continually emphasized that night-time sleep and daytime energy level can be determined by a number of factors in addition to one's subjective report of sleep adequacy. Such factors include overall emotional state (including degree of interest and level of motivation) and physical factors such as foods eaten and body rhythms (circadian, not astro-logical).

It must be emphasized time and again that different disci-plines profit from exposure to different points of view. And now as we turn, in our overview of the treatment of sleep-related dis-orders, to the nondrug approaches, both the neurochemists amongst us and the students of behavioral patterns and treatment methods can take advantage of the other's expertise to put to-gether coherent approaches to remedial intervention.

SLEEP HABITS

"Sleep hygiene" refers to the constructive attention paid to strategies which are conducive to promoting and permitting sleep. It includes the following rules of thumb with regard to difficulty sleeping:

- Make sure your bed, pillow, bed linens, and bed clothes are comfortable. By and large, a person's bed is the single most used piece of furniture in the house and it stands to reason that over time, one's mattress, like one's sneakers, may wear out, become less supportive, and needs to be replaced. The pillow should offer support, but if one is troubled by stom-ach or esophageal problems, like heartburn or reflux, medi-cal evaluation is mandatory first of all, and then raising the head of the bed by 10–15 degrees (rather than propping up with higher pillows and thereby buckling oneself at the waist) is indicated.

    With regard to bed clothes, a Vietnam veteran, victim of post-traumatic stress disorder (the new term for "shell shock") returned home and eventually recovered from his symptoms in every way except one. His sleep remained disturbingly light and insubstantial until it was suggested that he wear pajamas to sleep rather than remain, as he always had, in the nude. In psychotherapy sessions following this suggestion, a remarkable transformation occurred: first he began to speak of his feelings of vulnerability that pre-dated his war experience but were evoked by it; then he began to sleep more soundly, benefitting from the symbolic sense of security represented by the bed clothes he now wore.

- Make sure ambient temperature, noise and light are con-trolled if possible. In 1975, Japanese researchers reported that recordings of intrauterine sounds of maternal blood flow calmed newborn babies. Whether or not this finding will be replicated, the fact is that noise of the intensity of a vacuum cleaner does seem to induce sleep in newborns. It seems well-established that the use of "white noise" ma-chines, which generate a soothing, low intensity, rhyth-mically monotonous sound, can be useful in calming as well as masking potentially disruptive environmental disso-nance. Even Johann Sebastian Bach recognized that sound can soothe not only the savage beast, but the sleepless one as well: he wrote the "Goldberg Variations" to be played for insomniac royalty at bedtime.

- Unlike Louis XIV, one should use the bed only for sleep and sleep-compatible activities. If you cannot sleep within 30 minutes or so, get up and out of bed and engage in some diverting but nonstimulating activity (reading, TV, etc.). Do not watch the clock. Do not try too hard to fall asleep.

- Except in limited circumstances (for instance, in the rare situation of "over-tiredness"), discontinue all daytime naps (unless they are being used in the treatment of narcolepsy, as an alternative to psychostimulant medication). Certainly those after work or within 6 hours of bedtime should be stopped.

- Discontinue all sedatives and stimulants (including coffee, tea, caffeinated drinks, and chocolates). Discontinue alco-hol. If you smoke, do not do so right before bedtime. Do not eat a heavy meal less than 3 hours before bedtime, although light snacks or a soporific drink (like weak herbal tea) may be fine.

- Maintain a consistent schedule with regular sleeping and waking hours, regardless, 7 days a week. A clinical example of the potential effects of a chaotic, or at least inconsistent, schedule: Migraine headaches seem to be stimulated in many during REM sleep. Therefore, if a migraine-sufferer stays up late Friday night and then decides to sleep later into Saturday morning to make up for the relative sleep deprivation of his previous night's carousing, by lengthening his sleep cycle he will be exposed to more REM sleep-intensive time (the latter part of the sleep cycle, as you will recall) and thereby the propensity for an attack will be enhanced. Or alternatively: If during the weekend you try to make up for sleep loss, it is a little like the experience of jet lag, without the flying; you shift your sleep phase, tending to stay up later and later. Then, with the return of Monday and the work week's schedule demands, a disrupted sleep pattern, with perhaps some degree of sleep deprivation, has been established. And finally, regardless of when you go to bed, get up at the same time as always. Recognize that most sleep problems are the result of poor sleep habits.
- Perform only "quiet" activities before bedtime (reading, meditating, praying, relaxation or breathing exercises, bathing), and if such is not possible, allow some brief "cool down" time before getting into bed. If sleep does not seem imminent, consider whether there is some issue on your mind. If not, consider the possibility that, for whatever reason, you are not ready for sleep. Do not set unrealistic expectations for the amount of time you "should sleep." Instead, do something else and tell yourself that you will catch up on your sleep later, if necessary.
- Exercise only lightly, if at all, before bed. Light exercise, early in the evening, is felt by many to promote ease in falling asleep, a sense of deeper sleep, and a sense of well-being upon awakening. However, (and again it must be emphasized that simplistic conclusions are never warranted when dealing with systems as complex as the interface between human physiology and behavior) there are many components to the effect of exercise on sleep, including the baseline state of physical fitness. Specific details regarding a scheduling of effects and an outline of the correspondence

between the level of intensity and timing of exercise and the effects on the sleep–wake cycle remain to be determined. However, with regard to the effects of the type of physical activity in highly trained and "fit" athletes, it is clear that differences do exist based on the type of training that the athletes undergo. The aerobic, "endurance" training of the long-distance runner is associated with falling asleep more quickly, on average, with more NREM sleep components and a tendency to sleep longer than weight lifters with their "power" training. And, interestingly, athletes whose training includes both aerobic and power training exhibit dimensions of sleep patterns which are intermediate between these first two groups.

- If you snore excessively, seek professional evaluation, consider weight loss (if relevant), and do not sleep flat on your back. Depending on the type of sleep apnea that one suffers from, a number of interventions are possible, from tongue-retaining devices to be worn at night, to positive-pressure breathing devices and surgical correction of upper airway passages. Adjunctive medications may play some role as well, with agents used to affect the chemical balance in the blood that drives the brain's respiratory centers in central apnea, or agents used to increase the muscle tone surrounding the upper airway in obstructive apnea.

- Since patterns of sleep can be very personal, so too can be the remedies. With a willing partner, sexual activity can be a comfortable prelude to sleep, although not everyone at all times finds sex and orgasm a soporific. With sexual conflict and a rejecting partner, sleep may be a grudging refuge and retreat from unpleasant confrontation. In circumstances such as this, or with the presence of unremitting depression, anxiety or physical symptoms, professional help should be sought.

IS A SLEEP LAB FOR ME?

This has been a review of the range of "trouble-shooting" interventions possible for the spectrum of sleep-related disorders. It is not meant to be exhaustive, only suggestive. In fact, the entire book embodies an approach and philosophy which is "trouble-shooting." And if, after reading this, you find yourself as inter-ested in learning new facts as in acquiring a series of rituals to guide your sleep habits, my intentions will have been well-served.

Detailed exploration of all the specific treatment options currently available begins with a careful evaluation in which both the patient and the health-care professional form a cooperative investigative team. Ultimate referral to a sleep specialist or a sleep laboratory is indicated if, after thorough clinical assessment and preliminary intervention, a conservative approach has not worked, the need for special techniques (either evaluative like EEG and audiovisual recording under controlled circumstances, or thera-peutic like hypnosis, sleep restriction, scheduled exposure to bright light, and specialized pharmacotherapy) seems evident, or one suspects the presence of sleep apnea, nighttime seizures, periodic or daytime hypersomnia with functional impairment, or narcolepsy. And, of course, immediate evaluation should follow any sudden or devastating and persistent change in sleep–wake pattern.

One final note, going back to where it all began . . . our patterns of sleep established in childhood, not the Garden of Eden. What should parents do about a crying infant? Dr. Spock originally, and T. Berry Brazelton also, declared that a young child should be put to bed and left to cry himself or herself to sleep, to avoid "spoiling" the child. But, as Melvin Konner reported in an essay in the New York Times Magazine (1/8/89) entitled "Where Should Baby Sleep?" the Kung hunter–gatherers of Africa, as well as many mothers here, rejected the pediatricians' Spartan advice with observations along the lines of "They're not good little soldiers . . . they need to be favored . . . But they're only babies!" The handling of issues around a child's bedtime involves challeng-ing tasks for both the youngster and the parents. It raises issues of assessment and evaluation to new heights because of the inter-action among biology, personality, temperament, and environ-ment, because of the interwoven complex of developmental and family issues. You see, it is not that sleep problems necessarily start late in life . . . Twenty-five percent or more of children 1–4 years old have significant struggles around bedtime and about sleep. Suffice it to say that, although every case is different and that it is not possible to "spoil" the very young baby, a majority of persistent sleeping problems in children are consequences of inadvertently established parental procedures (like inconsistent handling of bedtime activities, permitting naps too close to bedtime, not allowing sufficient decompression transitional time in preparation for sleep, or reinforcing practices that prevent the child from learning to soothe himself or herself and thereby bring on sleep). Professional help is necessary to eliminate those practices supporting disruptive sleep patterns and to offer objective planning and support for the corrective behavioral interventions. These interventions are necessary and effective but demanding to implement and daunting.

Chapter 11

Wake Me Up When
It's Over
An Overview

THE RIVER OF CRYSTAL LIGHT

Andrew Borde wrote in praise of a balanced regimen of sleep, in the following terms:

> Sleep improved the digestion, refreshed the memory, nourished the blood . . . and comforted all the natural, animal, and spiritual powers. Immoderate sleep, on the other hand, moistened and lightened the brain, was bad for epilepsy and other infirmities of the head, hindered memory and quickness of wit, and perturbed the natural, animal and spiritual powers of man. Besides, immoderate sleep led to sinning, brevity of life, and displeased God.

This, written in 1576, in his postmedieval medical treatise entitled *A Compendious Regiment, or Dietarie of Health.*

As was mentioned in Chapter 1, Karl H. Dannenfeldt surveyed the theory and practice regarding sleep in the late Renaissance, and published his historical survey in 1986. From that study as well as other historical documentation, it becomes obvious that progress in man's understanding of the world around him often rests on a foundation built from fantasies and projections of how he thinks the world operates. As such, these constructs are in need of constant revision, as our data base and knowledge bank expand, and we come to incorporate more and more information into our world view.

With regard to sleep, Dannenfeldt canvassed the early medical thinking and the reasoning, at times tortuous, promulgated by early physicians attempting to understand the whys and wherefores of this phenomenon. From the first century Roman naturalist, Pliny, who wrote, in his *Natural History*, that anything that lacked a brain could not sleep, to the view of the Greek physician Galen (noted in his *On the Usefulness of the Parts of the Body*) that the brain was the repository of sensation and the source of all nerves, it is clear that early investigators were struggling with attempts to define and delineate not just the phenomenology of human behavior, but of the very interface between "body" and "psyche" itself. It was only later, in the late Renaissance, as Dannenfeldt points out, that anatomists, through meticulous although somewhat ingenuous dissections, determined that Aristotle, who had defined sleep as a suffering of the common sense, and who had held so much sway previously, was wrong in attributing nervous and sensory perception (and by extension, sleep) to the heart.

As primitive anatomical speculation gave way to somewhat more sophisticated anatomical observation, speculation then began again about less observable, less definable processes . . . processes underlying metabolism, growth, reproduction, and sleep. We have only recently written another chapter in this book of human investigation: with the advent of new technological electronic and electromagnetic probes (like the newly developed magnetoencephalography, which creates a picture of living brain tissue by detecting minute magnetic fields that are generated by neuronal cells in varying states of activity), with the discovery of adjunctive biochemicals useful as investigative tools within biological systems, with the development of new systems for detecting and analyzing the bewildering complexity of interactions in the biochemical "soup" within biological cells (like the high performance liquid chromatography, or HPLC, which can sort out, and therefore track, hundreds of different chemicals in biological specimens), with the development of more sophisticated means by which psychological phenomena may be observed and recorded, and with the creation of specific therapeutic agents which help to rectify biological systems gone awry and allow us to differentiate between the biological and psychological components of a system. It is within this context that this book has been an attempt to integrate and synthesize the varied research results, weaving them into a larger tapestry portraying the phenomenon of sleep, from what is known about it to what can go wrong with it. We have looked at some of the questions we all ask—why do some people remember their dreams, what are the consequences of changes in the amount of time we sleep, why is a brief nap refreshing for some and not for others. We have used a series of interlocking modules, giving us a way of thinking about fascinating, even "awesome," questions within the scientific medical tradition without having to resort to capricious or ritualistic thinking.

Clearly, many of the preceding paragraphs are speculative . . . informed, but speculative nonetheless. This speculation is not only fun, it also offers a challenge for further probing, for further inquiry and investigation. More like jazz than traditional western music, science relies on improvisation as new facts roll in at a rapid rate from all corners. Our focus on the human condition must involve far more than the traditional "humanistic" disciplines, or we risk being antihumanist! Once it was sufficient to say "nothing human is alien to me." At the risk of sounding grandiose, let us extend that concept to "nothing that we can learn about this universe is alien to us." As we recognize that plants have slow messenger systems in the form of hormones, some of which are directly relevant to us, we need not get maudlin and proclaim that "plants have feelings too." However, we would do well to appreciate what they have to teach us about ourselves. At the other extreme of the evolutionary pole, as we experiment with and fabricate "artificial brains" in the form of computers (very stupid at present, but learning at a prodigious pace), we may not merely be satisfied to congratulate ourselves on our unique human intelligence. Instead, we should learn more about ourselves from the very tools we fabricate. So the study of evolution, both the original biological kind and man's special technological kind, is relevant to all problems of a human scale, including the nature and origin of sleep.

As wonderful as our new insights regarding the workings of nature may be, the knowledge derived from our observations and investigations must be applied in an appropriate manner. A scientist's task is to distinguish between what is unique and what is commonplace, between what is a projection of our fantasy and what is materially "there," between what is insubstantial and what is substantial. Spurious conclusions can too easily be derived from wrong-headed, irrelevant or pseudoscientific attribution of an observed phenomenon to a look-alike, but otherwise quite dissimilar, phenomenon. Just like certain tests are designed for certain applications, particular facts are relevant to some but not all observations. For instance, even if you had had a wonderful experience driving a beautiful Rolls Royce across the country, from Los Angeles to New York City, you would still not be well-advised to reach the conclusion that . . . "since this is such a splendid machine, I think I'll just drive on to London!" As good a car as it may be the vehicle just wasn't made for the second leg of the trip.

Even though many of the mysteries of sleep (with its stream of internal tonic and clonic events) as well as many of the puzzles of waking life (with its own flow of external stimulus inputs and motor and prehensive activity) are beginning to yield to scientific inquiry, questions pertaining to the very nature and purpose of sleep, and to the effects of the types of sleep on waking performance, remain irresolute. We are able to sketch more definitively the interweaving of chemical messengers such as serotonin and the central nervous system regulation of functions such as mood level, eating behavior, pain responsiveness, and, of course, sleep. The curious fact that certain basic drives such as appetite, sex, and aggression can be heightened or diminished during depression has led to some interesting findings concerning a sexual arousal center in the brain. For example, a reduced level of serotonin in this center will lead to hypersexual behavior in many animals. It is interesting to note that cocaine has been found to reduce serotonin metabolism temporarily, and it certainly has a street reputation for aphrodisiac qualities. However, in humans, where dosage actually entering the brain cannot be accurately controlled, results are often contradictory. Again, timing, dosage, and setting are crucial to the net effect. Many people on antidepressant medication complain of decreased sex drive on higher doses and enhanced libido on lower ones. To what extent serotonin is the governing factor remains to be seen. But the focus of physical and psychological interplay in the organization and management of a behavioral phenomenon is what is important here.

BOTH SIDES OF THE LOOKING GLASS

An example of physical–behavioral interaction from an area other than that of sleep phenomena is further illustrative of this interplay. It pertains to the relatively recent discovery of androgen- and estrogen-sensitive areas in the brain. It has been possible to demonstrate dramatic effects from the prenatal administration of sex hormones on the physical size of these areas and the resultant quality of sexual functioning in the adult. More fascinating still is the influence of prenatal stress in demasculinizing rats by provoking a stress-related, premature peak in plasma testosterone that cannot be detected in the rat after birth. Here the principle of specific vulnerable growth periods, susceptible to the effects of external agents during a critical moment, and thereby affecting the course of subsequent development has broad applications in experimental animal studies. The application to humans is still tentative in many circumstances, but is worthy of serious consideration.

The final stage of basic gender identity formation would appear to be puberty, for most of us. Many hormonal balances are reworked at this time. A most dramatic example of the extent of this reworking is in children from a village in the Dominican Republic who, in rough translation, are known as "penis at thirteen." Due to an aberration in hormonal programming, these genetic boys seem to be girls at birth and are raised as such. However, at puberty a dramatic shift takes place with great enlargement of the shrunken penis and development of a full range of masculine characteristics. This is an extreme example, but more intermediate states exemplify the close interweaving of biological and psychological influences and effects.

FINAL COMMON PATHWAYS

Closer to the subject at hand, we know that the same midbrain nervous system neural circuits, known as the limbic system, are involved in the regulation of REM sleep as well as in the regulation of sexual, oral, and aggressive behavior. If this anatomical proximity provides the physical basis for a common bichemical mechanism controlling different physiological functions, then

Sigmund Freud intuited quite correctly that this physiological realm reflects this situation in a parallel fashion, when he observed how many different meanings can be condensed into one behavior. Here we have the suggestion of an underlying biochemical "final common pathway" subserving many different behavioral functions for the individual. Much like the arterial turnpike which provides a major access route for many different vehicles, with numerous purposes and different points of origin, and heading for various destinations, biochemical messenger routes provide access from and to many functional centers, carrying information of differing import depending, among other things, on patterns of transmission and structural intricacies of the receiving centers. Much of what is observed under the microscopic eye of the researcher in the minute dissection of a particular biological or psychological phenomenon must be understood as part of a mosaic, the overall pattern of which is what really matters. We must not lose ourselves within our own constrained perspective, unmindful of the contributions and insights of others. We are beginning to understand something of the chemical underpinnings of the neurological circuitry of certain biological systems. We are accomplishing this by proposing models of functioning and then testing these models for a reliable outcome. But whether our models are biochemical, cell-culture derived or the neural networks of computer simulation, we must remember that they are "models," attempts to understand and organize the known facts about an observed phenomenon, and, as an approximation, they are an organization of the facts observed, and should not be taken too literally.

Many basic questions remain open with regard to our understanding of a neuropsychobiological event such as sleep. How do neurons, firing their electrical impulses, convey "meaning"? How do changes in the connections among neural cell colonies translate into various reservoirs which both accumulate information and change over time? How can we bring data from a biological and physiological frame of reference and make this information more closely map on our understanding of the psychological reality of sleep? As an example, let us take the instance of the dream state. To again paraphrase the researcher Dr. Seymour Kety: We are beginning to develop a biochemistry of "dreaming," but not yet of "dreams."

In the process of searching for the center of sleep control in the brain, a number of factors representing possible chemical mechanisms controlling sleep have been found. These range from the neurotransmitters acteylcholine and glutamate, to chemical messengers called cytokines. These latter substances are involved in intercellular commerce and thereby provide a link between sleep, health, and disease, interacting as they do with that bulwark against disease known as the immune system. Additional chemical factors playing a role in the control of sleep phenomena are the hormones known as prostaglandins, which potentially provide a link between temperature- and sleep-regulation. We are just beginning to see clearly, for the first time, the intricate orchestration of multiple biological mechanisms, layered upon each other and interwoven by interdigitating biochemical systems.

And, then, as if this isn't enough, how are we to understand the additional layer of human existence added by psychological phenomena, and to integrate these events under a larger, chemo-neuro-behavioral umbrella? We have gone beyond the point where we have to be reminded that phenomena such as sleep, anesthesia, and coma, although all similar in appearance behaviorally, spring from different underlying circumstances occurring at the neuro-physiological level. We **now** must ask questions such as, how is experience transduced through organs of reception and perception (like the eye and the brain), to biochemical bases of reactivity and information storage. How, in other words, do we understand the functional continuity between protein molecules at the neuronal synapse and a subjective experience like devotion to family or love of The Beatles? At the center of this dizzying neuropsychobiological whirlpool is the sleep cycle, providing us with a slowly growing understanding of the biology of the regulation of psychological states . . . as well as, perhaps, of the affect of psychological states on biological functioning.

THE ELEPHANT AND THE BLIND MEN

Which brings us back to our journey's beginning: Earlier we spoke of the parable of the elephant and the blind men. The point was to emphasize the need, in one's search for knowledge, to be open to multiple perspectives. One of the main reasons for this relates to the principle of multideterminism, wherein a number of different functional components may be condensed into one agent, which is then modulated by various cofactors to selectively unleash its different functional subcomponent effects.

Look, for instance, at just one example of the sweepingly complex, multidetermined and broadly interactive functions that occur with serotonin. It represents just one of the many neuro-transmitters which affect neurochemical, neurophysiological and neuropsychological systems operating within the individual. From the regulation of sleep, appetite, mood, and sexual behaviors, to the control of anxiety states, obsessive–compulsive disorders, and suicidal behavior, to the disturbances in intellectual function-ing that accompanies schizophrenia and Alzheimers disease—serotonin has been implicated as a key neurochemical intermedi-ary in the expression of all of these phenomena.

Sigmund Freud was quite familiar with the principle of multi-determinism and, in fact, understood that "meaning" in dreams, as well as in other aspects of human psychological endeavor, was a specific example of this canon. As such, the search for under-standing of complex phenomena like "meaning," or anxiety, must be pursued from more than one perspective. For not only is nature parsimonious in that she uses actors on her stage in functionally economical ways, overlapping, and perhaps thereby masking, subtler functions by grosser ones, but also we mortals are ham-pered by our limited, individually secular views. We are, therefore, prohibited from the grander overview, except as, with their grad-ual accretion over time, many different observations congeal into one larger perspective. It is with respect to this process that the expression "the whole is greater than the sum of its parts" can then apply. The molecular biological insights of the present day are but extensions of the knowledge of previous decades regarding neu-roanatomy and neuroendocrinology. Our very awareness and aliveness, our sentiency, depends on interwoven systems in con-stant reciprocal contact with each other, governing equilibria among different shifting states. Our previously established under-standing of auditory physiology, reaction patterns and set-point sensitivities, for example, must now be combined with develop-ments on psychological frontiers for us to be able to begin to understand a phenomenon like the "love of Mozart."

Just as one must wary of a theorist who is elevated to the position of infallibility, one must likewise be wary of those who criticize creative thinkers solely from a political, axe-to-grind perspective. With regard to Freud, make no mistake. He was a perceptive innovator who, despite his culturally determined limitations and blindspots, was able to transcend the views of his day and approach a comprehension of the operation of the human psyche from a number of different vantage points which he attempted to unify into a coherent, larger, and ground-breaking theory. Often, opportunistic pop-psyche books which criticize his work reveal more about their lack of familiarity with his thinking, with the complexity of the tasks he wrestled with, and even with the nature of his personality and times, and less about the true and important deficits in his, admittedly, less-than-perfect theory. True, some equally limp-minded devotees established a cult-like dedication to his teachings, which they considered sacrosanct. But let us not cure such historic abuses of a discipline in its infancy by throwing out this proverbial baby with its accumulated bathwater! We can learn from all manner of human investigation, and we can profit from a synthesis of all manner of investigative pursuits. Even from the musings of the poet and playwright . . . like Shakespeare:

> "The innocent sleep,
> Sleep that knits up the ravell'd sleave of care
> The death of each day's life, sore labour's bath,
> Balm of hurt minds, great nature's second course,
> Chief nourisher of life's feast."
> *Macbeth* II, ii, 36–40

As we become more worldly-wise in our understanding of multideterminism and the relationships between body and mind, we begin to appreciate more fully the reciprocal connection between psychological distress and organic malady, and the fact that not all events looking the same turn out to be so. A case in point is the recent interest being given to an apparently newly delineated clinical entity dubbed "chronic fatigue syndrome." With regard to this "elephant," we have before us an overabundance of "blind sages." Depending on the specialty of the treating physician or the belief system of the provider of "alternative" medical care, a patient complaining of chronic fatigue may be diagnosed as suffering from one of a range of vaguely specified underlying physical disorders that presumably could account for the fatigue. These range from chronic, low-grade viral or fungal infections, to hypoglycemia, to a disorder called fibromyalgia, to chronic postnasal discharge, to sleep disorders.

It remains an open question as to the interrelationships among chronic fatigue, an individual's psychological profile, and sleep patterns, despite recent headlines claiming the pervasive but subtle presence of epidemic sleep deprivation among broad segments of our population. The fact that we are becoming increasingly aware of the role of sleep, and of biologically based cycles in general, is a further indicator of the progress of our knowledge. However, expect some sensationalism and perhaps overblown claims in the process of the information's trickle down from laboratory to public media. The fact that 84 conditions have recently been delineated as a new "International Classification of Sleep Disorders" is a testimony to our increasingly sophisticated and discriminating appreciation of this aspect of human physiology. We now look more closely at the practice of napping by the likes of Winston Churchill, Salvador Dali, Thomas Alva Edison, or Eleanor Roosevelt, and raise questions about the interrelationships among work schedules, sleep disorders, sense of well-being, and general productivity. While recognizing that for many insomniacs, napping is counterproductive, we are beginning to wonder whether, for the 25 percent or so of men and women who are on rotating work shifts, the cot and the self-timer will or should become just as much an office fixture as the water cooler and coffee dispenser have been.

Although the complaint of "poor sleep" is common, the **complaint** is not necessarily the same as the **fact** of poor sleep. Many who do have such complaints are not sleep-deprived at all but are suffering primary disorders of the sleep process. The current claim for the prevalence of environmentally demanded sleep deprivation is appealing because intermittent episodes of sleepiness are a common experience for us all. But additionally, this bandwagon is appealing to so many (professionals as well as lay persons) because in this early but growing state of our knowledge we have recognized an environmental contributor to a sleep problem about which something can be done! It is becoming increasingly clear that we do not just "adjust" to shift-induced disruptions in our cycles. We may, instead, become symptomatic and, in the case of sleep, accumulate a "debt" that needs to be restituted. It is here where we must begin to consider whether in fact the coffee machine or the nap room (giving new, or at least revitalized, meaning to the title "restroom") might better serve the purpose of workday rejuvenation, and whether the statistics suggesting higher incidence of ulcer and cardiac disease in workers on rotating shifts might not be better addressed by this new look at the workplace. Ultimately, we may discover that it is not so much that we are sleep-deprived. Rather, it may be that we have not appreciated the extent of our sensitivity to subtle but definite alterations in our daily rhythms, which affect our functioning and sense of health and contentment.

BIOLOGICAL RHYTHMS

It was back some 30 years ago when two researchers established the basis for the exploration of the cyclical rhythms of biology. From this initial work of Jurgen Aschoff and Colin Pittendrigh followed studies which recognized that many components of the psychology and physiology of many creatures are suffused with circadian rhythms. It became clear that, in mammals, these daily cycles were regulated by a central clock. This master "pacemaker" was determined to be located in that group of brain cells called the suprachiasmatic nucleus, which has intimate connections to the visual apparatus and which, in turn, is situated within a larger colony of brain cells, called the anterior hypothalamus. From this "clock" originates a recurrent orchestrating cycle of 24 hours (or close to it), as well as a process (called "entrainment") by which the clock and its attendant cycle can be fine-tuned to environmental alterations in light and other timing cues. Without the entrainment process, our "free-running" cycle time would be closer to 25 hours, perhaps reflecting something about the physical reality of the earth's rotation back at our evolutionary beginnings.

But mammals are not the only organisms that are keyed to cyclically recurrent schedules. The sleep of mammals, the rhythms of migratory birds, the reproduction cycles of insects, even the converging movements of swimming bacteria . . . all are examples of paced cycles of behavior. How are they effected? Through complex, intertwined systems from the sensory and physiological down to the chemical and molecular levels, and perhaps even further down to the electrical oscillations of nerve cells coupled into networks. And to what are they keyed? Ultimately, to aspects of their physical reality, like the light–dark cycle (called "photo-period"), like the movement of the tides, like alterations in temperature, like the multiyear periodicities characteristic of some climatic conditions. For life itself is not the only phenomenon noted for recurring cycles. And, finally, what can change, or reset, the clock? What affects its onset and what can change the peri-odicity of its cycle or of those ultradian ones influenced by it? These questions form the exciting basis for current research. Their answers will be gradually forthcoming over the next several years, as scientists attempt to understand the complexity of life's demands and the resultant multilayered and intricate response of the organism to these levies.

On a more subjective level, we know our lives in part by the personal benchmarks of our progress through the endless cycles of eternal time. At first we key ourselves to the cycles of day and night and the seasons. To this we add our rituals, religious as well as secular, and we follow the admonition of *Ecclesiastes* . . . "To everything there is a season and a time to every purpose under heaven . . ."

But as we become ever more technologically sophisticated, and even arrogant, we "fiddle," we "adjust," and we consequently "free" ourselves from the constraints of those cues we have been using to "time" ourselves. No longer are we limited in many of our activities by the unavailability of daylight. No longer are we held back by the harshest of a season's weather, be it in a sweltering tropical jungle or in a frigid arctic desert. No longer are we even constrained by the actual dates of memorial holidays that we ourselves constructed. We have rescheduled most of them to fall on Mondays!

"So," you may say, "more power to us!" Well, yes, but with regard to some of these manipulations, we forgot to take into account our biological wiring. Nature's clock is relatively unimpressed by the Johnny-come-lately tinkering of mankind. Our preoccupation with social needs and our disharmonious attempt to redefine certain innate cyclical qualities leave her apparently totally unmoved. She rules over a realm of inherent rhythms that go from growth and metabolism, to temperature, and immunological and circulatory regulating processes, and, further still, to behavioral cycles, in organisms ranging from simple multicellular plant life all the way up the phylogenetic scale, through insects, reptiles, birds, and mammals to man. We have to account, now, for the fact that a large percentage of births occur in the early morning hours, as do heart attacks. We must look at the report that most new Olympic records are established in the late afternoon hours. We must address the fact that man-made disasters like the Chernobyl, Three-Mile Island, Exxon Valdez, and Bhopal disasters occurred between the hours of 1:00 and 6:00 AM.

The fact that light, or, more formally, biologically active light, influences human circadian biorhythms significantly, can be demonstrated easily enough. Just blindfold subjects, or study the amplitudes of biological rhythms in blind individuals. The result will be a delay in rhythmic cycling in the former, and dampened excursion of the peaks and valleys of the cyclical excursions in the latter. Biologically active light is considered to be sunlight and intense, bright artificial light, not ordinary indoor light. Although many human bodily rhythms are entrained to time cues provided by daily and seasonal light–dark cycles, modern life with its use of artificial light removes many of these stimuli by effectively expanding the portion of these cycles during which high levels of activity can be maintained. This manipulation has the effect of raising social cues to a higher level of importance than the environmental light cues of earlier and simpler times.

What if we take it one step further: what if we attempt to manipulate previously entrained or perhaps "prewired" circadian rhythms by the use of intense artificial light. Experimental evidence suggests that after such exposure on two occasions each day for 5 days, normal volunteers' attention, concentration, reaction time, and sense of good sleep quality increases, and the number of nighttime awakenings decreases. If these same volunteers are exposed to partial sleep deprivation instead, they show the same increased sleep time and decreased midsleep awakenings, but their daytime performance suffers markedly. So we conclude that sleep and performance are interconnected, as are daylight and biological rhythms. Additional confounding data relates to the findings that sleep deprivation and biologically active light have both been reported to improve depression . . . suggesting, importantly enough, that depression may be more than just a disorder of mood.

But it becomes increasingly clear that numerous bodily structures and functions oscillate between maximal and minimal extremes, resonating to the harmonics of biological cycles and their pacemakers, and are keyed to hourly, daily, monthly, or yearly alterations in light, temperature, and other environmental stimuli. How news about the external environmental conditions and events is delivered to us through our perceptual apparatus and then transduced into information, transported by chemical messengers and electrical pulses to the central orchestrating conductors of our behavior in the brain, is the focus of much current investigation, but has yet to be established. The complexity of the mechanisms by which various circadian phenomena are interconnected, as well as the breadth of functions which fall within the bailiwick of these phenomena, however, has been established. It seems that functions ranging from inner core body temperature, to sleeping and eating, to thinking and performance may be marching to different internal drummers, and may go in and out of phase with respect to each other, episodically masking and dampening each other in complicated interwoven patterns in the process. We are just beginning to understand the consequences of altering the entrainment or synchronization of these rhythms. And with this recognition comes the realization that, just as there may be changes over an individual's lifetime with regard to his or her coordinated "symphony" of rhythms, there may also be differences between individuals with regard to their innate capacity to entrain their rhythms to shifts in external environmental cues or demands. We are on the threshold of a new understanding of mood disorders like depression and its relationship to disorders of sleep. We can also begin to understand why sleeping medications are not the panacea one might have expected them to be, although they do produce a short-term hypnotic effect pharmacologically, ultimately they may serve to disrupt and further desynchronize circadian or ultradian cycles. Finally, we may be on the verge of giving new meaning to the expression "I feel out of synch."

SLEEP AND MOOD

Psychiatrists, studying mental disorders of mood (the so-called affective disorders of mania and depression—from the word "affect" referring to emotion or feeling state) have noted that some patients seem to move through mood cycles irrespective of personal or environmental factors, as if driven by some internal "endogenous" engine. "Depression," however, is not a unitary phenomenon. Rather .it is a condition associated with diverse organic and behavioral components, and may represent a final common pathway (much like "fever") which can be reached from many different etiological or causative starting points. So, there are depressions which seem responsive to psychoactive antidepressant medication; others may be treated with sleep deprivation; and still others, called seasonal affective disorders, may be normalized by exposure to biologically active light (thereby given the lie to that old rock and roll refrain "Oh there ain't no cure for the summertime blues").

To the extent that we are better able to understand and describe the range of phenomena associated with sleep psychophysiology, to that extent we may be better able to understand the interplay among sleep, mood disturbances, and biorhythms. Whenever a physiological state, such as REM sleep, becomes more clearly described, correlations are sought between it and other states in the hope that the more intelligible phenomenon may serve as an investigative tool, illuminating a path which might lead toward understanding of the other, related, phenomenon. In the case of REM sleep, the disruption in sleep patterns of those suffering the agony of depression did not escape the attention of some sleep researchers.

In the flow of life, of growth, of change, one experiences, almost by definition, interactions, attachments . . . and painful losses. A hallmark of the reaction to loss in human beings is depression—a jarring sense of fragmentation accompanied by feelings of worthlessness, hopelessness, and helplessness, a withdrawal of interest and involvement with the outside world, and, often, certain physiological disruptions in eating and sleeping patterns.

It had been thought, following early observations, that there were certain tell-tale changes in sleep that occurred during depression. These included a shortened period of time between the individual's beginning to sleep and the onset of his first REM period. This shortening of "REM latency," coupled with an increased duration of the first REM period, and early and perhaps frequent awakenings, all seemed to suggest that REM sleep and depression may be interwoven in a way hitherto unsuspected. Since depression can be quite protean in its presentation, it was further hoped that these tell-tale changes might serve as a marker in those people in whom the depression itself was mild but the concomitant sleep changes were evident. Then, with a consistent methodology for measuring sleep patterns and their changes, we might be able to categorize and cluster different manifestations of the phenomenon, raise increasingly precise questions regarding causality, and address ourselves to treatment issues with a far greater sense of coherence and effectiveness.

Such was then the basis for the excitement surrounding the purported identification of a specific change in a sleep state associated with a specific behavioral state, depression. And, although answers to complex questions regarding the interface between human physiology and behavior do not come quickly, the work is in progress.

From another perspective, there were those investigators who, noting this covarying of sleep and depression, suggested that the increased REM sleep activity in depression reflected some increased "need" to dream. The reasoning was as follows: if dreaming time reflects time needed to consolidate information in an attempt to master the stresses and strains of living, a depressed person, struggling to master the slings and arrows of misfortune thrown his way, responds to an increased need for coping by increased dreaming time, just as a marathon runner responds to the demands of his challenge by assuming an appropriate state of increased physiological preparedness.

And from a third perspective still, some theorists proposed that the specific content of the depressed person's dreams might, by reflecting the status of self-esteem for instance, provide a clinically useful prognostic and monitoring tool for the treating doctor. Some of these suggestions are more poetic and less empirically substantiated at this point in time, yet all are of interest. But in considering the overlapping of sleep phenomena and mood disorder, we must also consider the possibility that, more generally, a disorder in the coordination of the body's biological rhythm orchestra, or, more specifically, the REM cycle gone awry, underlie the phenomenology of depression. This hypothesis suggests that alterations in REM sleep may not be a consequence of depression, but rather, may reflect an underlying dysregulation of bio-synchronicity. The disruption in biorhythms, then, results in a disruption of REM sleep characteristics and a psychological state (of dysphoria, malaise . . . feeling lousy) which is the subjective concomitant of physiological systems gone wrong.

To the extent that we become increasingly competent at delineating the alterations and vagaries of sleep psychophysiology, to that extent do we come closer to using the monitoring of sleep as one more effective measure of central nervous system function and integrity, and come one step closer to understanding human existence from both sides of the looking glass, the mind and the brain. To the extent that we see reasoned skepticism, investigation, and knowledge as the beacon to illuminate our path, to that extent do we follow a surer path to a broader horizon.

Bibliography

CHAPTERS 1 AND 2

Berger, R. J., "Slow Wave Sleep, Shallow Torpor and Hibernation: Homologous States of Diminished Metabolism and Body Temperature," *Biological Psychology* **19**:305–326, 1984.

Campbell, S. S. & Tobler, I., "Animal Sleep: A Review of Sleep Duration Across Phylogeny," *Neuroscience & Biobehavioral Reviews* **8**:269–300, 1984.

Cole, K. C., *Sympathetic Vibrations, Reflections on Physics as a Way of Life*, William Morrow & Co., N.Y., 1985.

Dannenfeldt, K. H., "Sleep: Theory and Practice in the Late Renaissance," *Journal of History of Medicine & Allied Sciences* **41**:415–441, 1986.

Davis, M., Jacobs, B. L. & Schoenfeld, R. I. (eds.), "Modulation of Defined Vertebrate Neural Circuits," *Annals of the New York Academy of Science* **563**:1–195, 1989.

Dement, W. C., "A Personal History of Sleep," *Journal of Clinical Neurophysiology* **7(1)**:17–47, 1990.

Hawkins, D. R., "Dreaming, Neurobiology and Psychoanalysis," *Psychiatric Annals* **20(5)**:238–244, 1990.

Haydu, G. G. (ed.), "Patterns of Integration from Biochemical to Behavioral Processes," *Annals of the New York Academy of Science* **193**:1–310, 1972.

Hobson, A. J., *Sleep*, Scientific American Library, N. Y., 1989.

Ishihara, K., Miyasita, A., Inugami, M. *et al.*, "Differences in Sleep–Wake Habits between Active Morning and Evening Subjects," *Sleep* **10(4)**:330–342, 1987.

Johnson, L. C., "Are Stages of Sleep Related to Waking Behavior?" *American Scientist* **61**:326–338, 1973.

Koella, W. P., "A Partial Theory of Sleep. A Novel View of Its Phenomenology and Organization," *European Neurology* **25 (Suppl. 2)**:9–17, 1986.

Luce, G. G. & Segal, J., *Sleep*, Lancer, N.Y., 1966.

Rechtschaffen, A., Bergmann, B. M., Everson, C. A., et al., "Sleep Deprivation in the Rat: Conceptual Issues," Sleep **12(1)**:1–4, 1989.

Rosenblatt, A. D. & Thickstun, J. T., Modern Psychoanalytic Concepts in a General Psychology, Psychological Issues Vol. XI, Nos. 2/3, Monograph 42/43, International University Press, N.Y., 1977.

Sagan, C., Broca's Brain, Ballantine Books, N.Y., 1978.

Sidman, M., Tactics of Scientific Research, Basic Books Inc., N.Y., 1960.

Vieth, J., "Vigilance, Sleep and Epilepsy," European Neurology **25(Suppl. 2)**:128–133, 1986.

Walker, J. M., Garber, A., Berger, R. J., et al., "Sleep and Estivation," Science **204**:1098–1100, 1979.

CHAPTER 3

Adam, K., Tomeny, M. & Oswald, I., "Physiological and Psychological Differences between Good and Poor Sleepers," Journal of Psychiatric Research **20(4)**:301–316, 1986.

Binkley, S., Tome, M. B. & Mosher, K., "Weekly Phase Shifts of Rhythms Self-reported by Almost Feral Human Students," Physiology & Behavior **46**:423–427, 1989.

Bixler, E. O. & Vela-Bueno, A., "Normal Sleep: Patterns and Mechanisms," Seminars in Neurology **7(3)**:227–235, 1987.

Bonnet, M. H. & Rosa, R. R., "Sleep and Performance in Young Adults and Older Normals and Insomniacs during Acute Sleep Loss and Recovery," Biological Psychology **25**:153–172, 1987.

Borbely, A. A., "A Two Process Model of Sleep Regulation," Human Neurobiology **1**:195–204, 1982.

Brissette, S., Montplaisir, J., Godbout, R. et al., "Sexual Activity and Sleep in Humans," Biological Psychiatry **20**:758–763, 1985.

Campbell, S. S., Gillin, J. C., Kripke, D. F. et al., "Gender Differences in the Circadian Temperature Rhythms of Healthy Elderly Subjects," Sleep **12(6)**: 529–536, 1989.

Czeisler, C., Rios, C., Sanchez, R. et al., "Phase Advance and Reduction in Amplitude of the Endogenous Circadian Oscillator Correspond with Systematic Changes in Sleep–Wake Habits and Daytime Functioning in the Elderly," Sleep Research **15**:268, 1986.

Fisher, B. E., Poulers, C. & McGuire, K., "Children's Sleep Behavioral Scale," Perceptual & Motor Skills **68**:227–236, 1989.

Foret, J., Touron, N., Clodore, M. et al., "Modifications of Sleep Structure by Brief Forced Awakenings at Different Times of the Night," Electroencephalography & Clinical Neurophysiology **75**:141–147, 1990.

Goodman, J., Radomski, M., Hart, L. et al., "Maximal Aerobic Exercise Following Prolonged Sleep Deprivation," International Journal of Sports Medicine **10**:419–423, 1989.

Hobson, J. A., Spagna, T. & Malenka, R., "Ethology of Sleep Studied with Time-lapse Photography: Postural Immobility and Sleep-cycle Phase in Humans," *Science* **201(29)**:1251–1253, 1978.

Moore-Ede, M. C., Weitzman, E., Kronauer, C., & Czeisler, C., "Physiology of the Circadian Timing System: Predictive Versus Reactive Homeostasis," *American Journal of Physiology* **250(5 Pt. 2)**:R737–752, 1986.

Morgan, K., Healey, D. W. & Healey, P. J., "Factors Influencing Persistent Subjective Insomnia in Old Age," *Age & Ageing* **18**:117–122, 1989.

Reynolds III, C. F., Kuppfer, D. J., Hoch, C. C. *et al.*, "Sleep Deprivation in Healthy Elderly Men and Women: Effects on Mood and on Sleep During Recovery," *Sleep* **9(4)**:492–501, 1986.

Strauch, I. & Meier, B., "Sleep Need in Adolescents," *Sleep* **11(4)**:378–386, 1988.

Thorpy, M. J., Korman, E., Spielman, A. J. *et al.*, "Delayed Sleep-Phase Syndrome in Adolescents," *Journal of Adolescent Health Care* **9**:22–27, 1988.

CHAPTER 4

Ambrosini, M. V., Sadile, A. G., Gironi Carnevale, U. A., *et al.*, "The Sequential Hypothesis on Sleep Function," *Physiology & Behavior* **43**:325–337, 1988.

Breland, K., & Breland, M., *Animal Behavior*, MacMillan Co., N.Y., 1968.

Davis, B. D., "Sleep and the Maintenance of Memory," *Perspectives in Biology & Medicine* **28(3)**:457–464, 1985.

Dimond, S. J. & Blizard, D. A. (eds.), "Evolution and Lateralization of the Brain," *Annals of the New York Academy of Science* Vol. 299, 1977.

Dinges, D. F., Orne, M. T., Whitehouse, W. G., *et al.*, "Temporal Placement of a Nap for Alertness," *Sleep* **10(4)**:313–329, 1987.

Fagioli, I., Cipolli, C. & Tuozzi, G., "Accessing Previous Mental Sleep Experience in REM and NREM Sleep," *Biological Psychology* **29**:27–38, 1989.

Foulkes, D., Bradley, L., Cavallero, C., *et al.*, "Processing of Memories and Knowledge in REM and NREM Dreams," *Perceptual and Motor Skills* **68**:365–366, 1989.

Friedman, R. C., Biggar, J. T., & Kornfeld, D. S., "The Intern and Sleep Loss," *New England Journal of Medicine* **285**:201–203, 1971.

Gabel, S., "Information Processing in REMS," *Journal of Nervous and Mental Disease* **175(4)**:193–200, 1987.

Gordon, H. W. & Stoffer, D. S., "Ultradian Rhythms of Right and Left Hemisphere Function," *International Journal of Neuroscience* **47**:57, 1989.

Harsh, J., Badia, P., O'Rourke, D. *et al.*, "Factors Related to Behavioral Control by Stimuli Presented During Sleep," *Psychophysiology* **24(5)**:535–541, 1987.

Holden, C. (ed.), "Leonardo's Secret: Cat Naps," *Science* **249**:244, 1990.

Kepler, T. B., Marder, E. & Abbott, L. F., "The Effect of Electrical Coupling on the Frequency of Model Neuronal Oscillators," *Science* **248**:83–86, 1990.

Siegel, J. M., "Mechanisms of Sleep Control," *Journal of Clinical Neurophysiology* **7(1)**:49–65, 1990.

Vygotsky, L. S., *Thought and Language*, MIT Press, Cambridge, Mass., 1962.

CHAPTER 5

Bonner, M. H., "Effect of Sleep Disruption on Sleep, Performance and Mood," *Sleep* **8(1):**11–19, 1985.

Bramham, C. R. & Bolek, S., "Synaptic Plasticity in the Hippocampus is Modulated by Behavioral State," *Brain Research* **493:**75–86, 1989.

Crick, F. & Mitchison, G., "The Function of Dream Sleep," *Nature* **304:**111–114, 1983.

Gillin, J. C., Buchsbaum, M. S., Jacobs, L. S., *et al.*, "Partial REM Sleep Deprivation, Schizophrenia and Field Articulation," *Archives of General Psychiatry* **30:**653–657, 1974.

Guerrien, A., Dujardin, K., Mandai, O., *et al.*, "Enhancement of Memory by Auditory Stimulation During Postlearning REMS in Humans," *Physiology & Behavior* **45:**947–950, 1989.

Hennevin, E., Hars, B., & Bloch, V., "Improvement of Learning by Mesencephalic Reticular Stimulation during Postlearning Paradoxical Sleep," *Behavioral & Neural Biology* **51:**291–306, 1989.

Hook, S. (ed.), *Dimensions of Mind*, Collier Books, N.Y., 1961.

Horne, J., *Why We Sleep*, Oxford University Press, N.Y., 1988.

Jacques, C. H. M., Lynch, J. C. & Samkoff, J. S., "The Effects of Sleep Loss on Cognitive Performance of Resident Physicians," *Journal of Family Practice* **30(2):**223–229, 1990.

Johnson, L. C., "Sleep Deprivation and Performance," *in* W. B. Webb (ed.), *Biological Rhythms, Sleep & Performance*, pp. 111–141, Wiley, Chichester, U.K., 1982.

Jaynes, J., *The Origin of Consciousness in the Breakdown of the Bicameral Mind*, Houghton Mifflin Co., Boston, Massachusetts, 1976.

Lydic, R., "State-dependent Aspects of Regulatory Physiology," *FASEB Journal* **1:**6–15, 1987.

Science (report), **249:**244, 1990.

Trinder, J., Montgomery, I. & Paxton, S. J., "The Effect of Exercise on Sleep: The Negative View," *Acta Physiologica Scandinavica* **133 (Suppl. 574):**14–20, 1988.

Udin, S. B. & Scherer, W. J., "Restoration of the Plasticity of Binocular Maps by NMDA." *Science* **249:**669–671, 1990.

Vuori, I., Urponen, H., Hasan, J. *et al.*, "Epidemiology of Exercise Effects on Sleep," *Acta Physiologica Scandinavica* **133 (Suppl. 574):**3–7, 1988.

CHAPTER 6

de Saint Hilaire-Kafi, Z., Depoortere, H. & Nicolaidis, S., "Does Cholecystokinin Induce Physiological Satiety and Sleep?", *Brain Research* **488:**304–310, 1989.

Kolata, G. B., "Brain Biochemistry: Effects of Diet," *Science* **192:**41–42, 1976.

Medsger, Jr., T. A., "Tryptophan-induced Eosinophilia-myalgia Syndrome" (Editorial), *New England Journal of Medicine* **322(13):**926–927, 1990.

Peirano, P., Fagioli, I., Singh, B. B. *et al.*, "Effect of Early Human Malnutrition on Waking and Sleep Organization," *Early Human Development* **20:**67–76, 1989.

Singh, M. M. & Kay, S. R., "Wheat Gluten as a Pathogenic Factor in Schizophrenia," *Science* **191**:401–402, 1976.

Williams, R. L. & Karacan, I. (eds.), *Pharmacology of Sleep*, John Wiley & Sons, N.Y., 1976.

Wurtman, R. J. & Wurtman, J. J. (eds.), *Nutrition and the Brain, Volumes 1 and 2*, Raven Press, N.Y., 1977.

CHAPTER 7

Barlow, Jr., R. B., "What the Brain Tells the Eye," *Scientific American* **262**:90–95, 1990.

Doran, A. R., Labarca, R., Wolkowitz, O. M., *et al.*, "Circadian Variation of Plasma HVA Levels is Attenuated by Fluphenazine in Patients with Schizophrenia," *Archives of General Psychiatry* **47**:558–562, 1990.

Dube, S., Jones, D. A., Bell, J., *et al.*, "Interface of Panic and Depression: Clinical and Sleep EEG Correlates," *Psychiatric Research* **19**:119–133, 1986.

Lewy, A. J., "Treating Chronobiologic Sleep and Mood Disorders with Bright Light," *Psychiatric Annals* **17(10)**:664–668, 1987.

Livermore, Jr., A. H. & Stevens, J. R., "Light Transducer for the Biological Clock: A Function for REM," *Journal of Neural Transmission* **72**:37–42, 1988.

Parry, B. L., Mendelson, W. B., Duncan, W. C., *et al.*, "Longidutinal Sleep EEG, Temperature and Activity Measurements Across the Menstrual Cycle in Patients with Premenstrual Depression and in Controls," *Psychiatric Research* **30**:285–303, 1989.

Ralph, M. R., Foster, R. G., Davis, F. C., *et al.*, "Transplanted Suprachiasmatic Nucleus Determines Circadian Period," *Science* **247**:975–978, 1990.

Rusak, B., Robertson, H. A., Wisden, W., *et al.*, "Light Pulses that Shift Rhythms Induce Gene Expression in the Suprachiasmatic Nucleus," *Science* **248**:1237–1239, 1990.

Sack, D. A. & Wehr, T. A., "Circadian Rhythms in Affective Disorders," *in* Georgotas, A. & Cancro, R. (eds), *Depression and Mania*, Elsevier, N.Y., 1988.

Sitaram, N., Moore, A. M., & gillin, J. C., "Experimental Acceleration and Slowing of REM Sleep Ultradian Rhythm," *Nature* **274**:490–492, 1978.

Vertes, R. P., "A Life-sustaining Function for REM Sleep: A Theory," *Neuroscience & Biobehavioral Reviews* **10**:371–376, 1986.

Wu, J. C. & Bunney, W. E., "The Biological Basis of an Antidepressant Response to Sleep Deprivation and Relapse," *American Journal of Psychiatry* **147(1)**:14–21, 1990.

CHAPTER 8

Bergmann, M. S., "The Intrapsychic and Communicative Aspects of the Dream," *International Journal of Psycho-Analysis* **47**:356–363, 1966.

Brenner, C., "Dreams in Psychoanalytic Practice," *Journal of Nervous & Mental Disease* **149**:122, 1969.

Foulkes, D. & Vogel, G., "The Current Status of Laboratory Dream Research," *Psychiatric Annals* **4**:12, 1974.

Freud, S., *The Interpretation of Dreams* (Strachey, J., trans. & ed.), Avon Books, N.Y., 1969.

Hartmann, E. L., "The D-State," *New England Journal of Medicine* **273(1)**:30–34, 1965, & *New England Journal of Medicine* **273(2)**:87–92, 1965.

Hobson, J. A. & McCarley, R. W., "The Brain as a Dream State Generator: An Activation-Synthesis Hypothesis of the Dream Process," *American Journal of Psychiatry* **134**:1335–1348, 1977.

Jones, R. M., "The Psychoanalytic Theory of Dreaming—1968," *Journal of Nervous & Mental Disease* **147(6)**:587–604, 1968.

Koulack, D., Prevost, F. & De Koninck, J., "Sleep, Dreaming and Adaptation to Stressful Intellectual Activity," *Sleep* **8(3)**:244–253, 1985.

Miller, L., "On the Neuropsychology of Dreams," *Psychoanalytic Review* **76(3)**:375–401, 1989.

Snyder, F., "Toward an Evolutionary Theory of Dreaming," *American Journal of Psychiatry* **123**:121–130, 1966.

Ullman, M. & Limmer, C. (eds.), *The Variety of Dream Experience*, Continuum, N.Y., 1987.

Vogel, G. W., "An Alternative View of the Neurobiology of Dreaming," *American Journal of Psychiatry* **135(12)**:1531–1534, 1978.

Wheelis, A., *How People Change*, Harper & Row, N.Y., 1973.

Whitman, R. M., Kramer, M., Ornstein, H., *et al.*, "The Physiology, Psychology and Utilization of Dreams," *American Journal of Psychiatry* **124(3)**:287–302, 1967.

Winson, J., *Brain Psyche: The Biology of the Unconscious*, Anchor/Doubleday, N.Y., 1985.

Wright, J. & Koulack, D., "Dreams and Contemporary Stress: A Disruption-avoidance-adaptation Model," *Sleep* **10(2)**:172–179, 1987.

CHAPTER 9

Aldrich, M. S., "Narcolepsy," *New England Journal of Medicine* **323(6)**:389–394, 1990.

American Psychiatric Association, *DSM-III, Diagnostic and Statistical Manual of Mental Disorders*, APA, Wash., D.C., 1987.

Barabas, G., Ferrari, M. & Matthews, W. S., "Childhood Migraine and Somnambulism," *Neurology* **33**:948–1048, 1983.

Broughton, R. J., "Sleep Disorders: Disorders of Arousal?", *Science* **159(3819)**:1070–1078, 1968.

Chase, M. H. & Morales, F. R., "Subthreshold Excitatory Activity and Motorneuron Discharge During REM Periods of Active Sleep," *Science* **221**:1195–1198, 1983.

Coleman, R. M., *Wide Awake at 3:00 A.M.*, W. H. Freeman & Co., N.Y., 1986.

Connell, H. M., Persley, G. V. & Sturgess, J. L., "Sleep Phobia in Middle Childhood," *Journal of the American Academy of Child and Adolescent Psychiatry* **26(3)**:449–452, 1987.

Editorial, *The Lancet,* pp. 925–926, "Snoring and Sleepiness" Oct. 26, 1985.

Ely, D. L. & Mostardi, R. A., "The Effect of Recent Life Stress, Life Assets, and Temperament Pattern on CV Risk Factors for Akron City Police," *Journal of Human Stress* **12**:77–91, 1986.

Fukuda, K., Miyasita, A., Inugami, M., *et al.,* "High Prevalence of Isolated Sleep Paralysis," *Sleep* **10(3)**:279–285, 1986.

Gillin, J. C. & Byerley, W. F., "The Diagnosis and Management of Insomnia," *New England Journal of Medicine* **322(4)**:239–248, 1990.

Kales, J. D., Soldatos, C. R., & Kales, A., "Treatment of Sleep Disorders," *Psychiatric Medicine* **4(2)**:209–227, 1987.

Kleitman, N., "The Basic Rest-Activity Cycle—22 Years Later," *Sleep* **5**:311–317, 1983.

Lydic, R. & Biebuyck, J. F. (eds.), *Clinical Physiology of Sleep,* American Physiological Society, Bethesda, Maryland, 1988.

Mahowald, M. W., Bundlie, S. R., Hurwitz, T. D., *et al.,* "Sleep Violence—Forensic Science Implications," *Journal of Forensic Science* **35(2)**:413–432, 1990.

Manfredi, R. L., Vgontzas, M. D. & Kales, A., "An Update on Sleep Disorders," *Bulletin of the Menninger Clinic* **53(3)**:250–273, 1989.

Mellman, T. A. & Uhde, T. W., "Sleep Panic Attacks: New Clinical Findings and Theoretical Implications," *American Journal of Psychiatry* **146(9)**:1204–1207, 1989.

Moore-Ede, M. C. & Richardson, G. S., "Medical Implications of Shift Work," *Annual Review of Medicine* **36**:607–617, 1985.

Oswald, I. & Adam, K., "Rhythmic Raiding of Refrigerator Related to REM," *British Medical Journal* **292**:589, 1986.

Roffwarg, H. & Erman, M., "Evaluation and Diagnosis of the Sleep Disorders," *in* R. C. Hales & A. J. Frances (eds.), *American Psychiatric Association Annual Review, Volume 4,* pp. 294–328, APA Press, Washington, D.C., 1985.

Sahota, P. K. & Dexter, J. D., "Sleep and Headache Syndromes," *Headache* **30**:80–84, 1990.

Siegel, J. M., Nienhuis, R., Fahringer, H. M. *et al.,* "Neuronal Activity in Narcolepsy: Identification of Cataplexy-Related Cells in the Medial Medulla," *Science* **252**:1315–1318, 1991.

Thach, B. T., "Sleep Apnea in Infancy and Childhood," *Medical Clinics of North America* **69(6)**:1289–1315, 1985.

Thorpy, M. J., "Classification of Sleep Disorders," *Journal of Clinical Neurophysiology* **7(1)**:67–81, 1990.

Turino, G. M. & Goldring, R. M., "Sleeping and Breathing" (editorial), *New England Journal of Medicine* **299(18)**:1009–1010, 1978.

Williams, R. L., Karacan, I. & Moore, C. A. (eds.), *Sleep Disorders Diagnosis & Treatment,* Wiley Interscience, N.Y., 1988.

Wooten, V., "Evaluation and Management of Sleep Disorders in the Elderly," *Psychiatric Annals* **20(8)**:466–470, 1990.

Zuckerman, B., Stevenson, J. & Bailey, V., "Sleep problems in Early Childhood," *Pediatrics* **80(5)**:664–670, 1987.

CHAPTER 10

Borbely, A. A. & Tobler, I., "Endogenous Sleep-Promoting Substances and Sleep Regulation," *Physiology Review* **69(2)**:605–661, 1989.

Carskadon, M. A., Dement, W. C., Mitler, M. M., Guilleminault, C. *et al.*, "Self-reports Vs. Sleep Lab Findings in 122 Drug-free Subjects with Complaints of Chronic Insomnia," *American Journal of Psychiatry* **133(12)**:1382–1388, 1976.

Czeisler, C. A., Johnson, M. P., Duffy, J. F. *et al.*, "Exposure To Bright Light and Darkness To Treat Physiologic Maladaptation To Night Work," *New England Journal of Medicine* **322**:1253–1259, 1990.

Ferber, R., "Sleep, Sleeplessness, and Sleep Disruptions in Infants and Young Children," *Annals of Clinical Research* **17**:227–234, 1985.

Gillin, J. C. & Byerley, W. E., "The Diagnosis and Treatment of Insomnia," *New England Journal of Medicine* **322**:239–248, 1990.

Jurado, J. L., Fernandez-Mas, R. & Fernandez-Guardiola, A., "Effects of 1 Week Administration of 2 Benzodiazepines on the Sleep and Early Daytime Performance of Normal Subjects," *Psychopharmacology* **99**:91–93, 1989.

Keener, M. A., Zeanah, C. H. & Anders, T. A., "Infant Temperament, Sleep Organization and Nighttime Parental Interventions," *Pediatrics* **81(6)**:762–771, 1988.

Mendelson, W. B., "The Search For The Hypnogenic Center," *Progress in Neuro-Psychopharmacology & Biological Psychiatry* **14**:1–12, 1990.

Pasche, B., Erman, M. & Mitler, M., "Letters to the Editor," *New England Journal of Medicine* **323(7)**:486–487, 1990.

Prinz, P. N., Vitiello, M. V., Raskind, M. A. & Thorpy, M. J., "Geriatrics: Sleep Disorders and Aging," *New England Journal of Medicine* **323(8)**:520–527, 1990.

Richman, N., Douglas, J., Hunt, H. *et al.*, "Behavioural Methods in the Treatment of Sleep Disorders," *Journal of Clinical Psychology & Psychiatry* **26(4)**:581–590, 1985.

Rickert, V. I. & Johnson, C. M., "Reducing Nocturnal Awakening and Crying in Infants and Young Children," *Pediatrics* **81(2)**:203–211, 1988.

CHAPTER 11

Brown, N. O., *Life Against Death*, Wesleyan University Press, Middletown, Connecticut, 1959.

Index